ACCLAIM FOR MICHAEL THURMOND'S PREVIOUS BOOK

6 day BODY MAKEOVER

"He is a true master of his craft . . . pragmatic, determined, and even dogged in his determination to succeed for his clients. His results never fail to astonish me."
—Jon A. Perlman, MD, FACS, clinical assistant professor of plastic surgery at UCLA Medical Center

"Thurmond has developed a body type blueprinting system that allows readers to customize their diet regimen . . . Thurmond also gives fat-burning, low-intensity exercises to help lose weight and keep it off."
—*Toronto Star*

"A diet plan with staying power. [From dieter] Dolores Thompson, 'It worked for me! It's been six years and counting. I even became a personal trainer!'"
—*First for Women Magazine*

"A wealth of sound information."   **—MonstersandCritics.com**

"This book is packed with sensible tips and good advice . . . The book is written in a very accessible, easy-to-use style, with information presented in a clear, straightforward way."   **—*Berkshire Eagle* (MA)**

"Thurmond has menus and serving sizes all mapped out . . . sound weight reduction advice with quick and safe results."   **—BookLoons.com**

"Based on sound principles that just make sense about the body. Additionally, Michael gives you a 'what's next' after his *6-Day Body Makeover* with valuable tips to get you going and keep you on target."   **—Review-Books.com**

12 day BODY SHAPING MIRACLE

Change Your Shape, Transform Problem Areas, and Beat Fat for Good

MICHAEL THURMOND

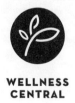

WELLNESS CENTRAL

NEW YORK   BOSTON

Wellness Central
Hachette Book Group USA
237 Park Avenue
New York, NY 10017

Visit our Web site at www.HachetteBookGroupUSA.com.

Printed in the United States of America
Originally published in hardcover by Hachette Book Group USA.
First Trade Edition: March 2008
10 9 8 7 6 5 4 3 2 1

Wellness Central is an imprint of Grand Central Publishing.
The Wellness Central name and logo is a trademark of Hachette Book Group USA, Inc.

The Library of Congress has catalogued the hardcover edition as follows:
Thurmond, Michael, personal trainer .
     The 12 day body shaping miracle : change your shape, transform problem areas, beat fat for good / by Michael Thurmond. — 1st ed.
         p. cm.
     Summary: "On the heals of his National bestseller, television body makeover specialist Michael Thurmond helps readers transform their body shape in just 12 days with his workout program"— Provided by the publisher.
     ISBN–13 : 978-0-446-52766-8
     ISBN–10 : 0-446-52766-1
  1. Exercise. 2. Nutrition. I. Title.
     RA781.T48 2007
     613.7'1- -dc22

                                                                        2006019165

     ISBN 978-0-446-69827-6 (pbk.)

Book design and text composition by HRoberts Design

To my wonderful clients and readers, and the millions of people who are using my
makeover programs to reshape their bodies and transform their health.
May you take the information in this book and be the best you've ever been!

ACKNOWLEDGMENTS

i feel so fortunate, so humble, and so grateful to have so many talented people around me.

Once again, my deepest appreciation goes to Jeff Clifford, Brady Caverly, and Lenny Sands, all of Provida Life Sciences, who have played such a huge role in bringing my makeover programs to the attention of the world through three hit infomercials. This Provida team, with skilled insight, creativity, and ingenuity, took my basic approach to reshaping the human body and turned it into a phenomenal product called Michael Thurmond's *6-Week Body Makeover,* now one of the most popular and successful weight-loss and exercise programs available. Provida's work and proven ability at product development and marketing have been a true springboard for me and, more than that, have enabled millions of people to achieve their dream bodies.

Three other key people at Provida, Dolores Thompson, Paul Duff, and Matt Vance, must also be thanked for their help in coordinating key aspects of this book, and most of all for helping inspire the millions of people who have learned how to make over their bodies using my techniques.

My agent, Barbara Lowenstein, is among the most dynamic in the literary world. This is our second book together, and I hope that there will be many more. Thank you so much.

My creative expert and friend, Maggie Greenwood-Robinson, PhD, was an enormous help to me. Maggie is a real pro at organization, creativity, editing, and collaboration. Plus, she was able to keep up with me in the gym when I taught her my body-shaping techniques. Thank you so much for your infectious enthusiasm and can-do spirit.

Thanks to my Warner Books team, Diana Baroni, Natalie Kaire, and Leila Porteous, whose input, direction, coordination, and hardworking support were invaluable to this undertaking. I appreciate all of you so much.

My anchor in life, Benita Heet, oversees just about every aspect of my life and does so with incredible efficiency, grace, and dedication. Because of you, my life has changed for the better.

Thankful appreciation to Kris Reid, who was my right-hand man on ABC's *Extreme Makeover* and who manages my company as if it were his own, a rare and valuable trait. A special thanks to Juan Perez, my vice president, who has been through the ups and downs of an "overnight" success.

Thanks go to my terrific staff. You are the best! Each of you gives of yourself every single day to help people everywhere achieve better health and well-being. A special mention to Leah Hyman and Nicole Rollolazo, who are two of my incredible trainers and the exercise models for this book. To Alisa Daglio, who manages our Spa Body Makeover program, and our splendid staff there—who all work efficiently to ensure that our spa clients are happy and informed, and leave with a whole new body and lifestyle—thank you.

And finally, to all my wonderful clients: I could not have done what I do without you. Thank you for trusting me to guide you through your journey to discovering how to look and feel your best at all times.

CONTENTS

INTRODUCTION

Time Is Prime: Just Give Me 12 Days!

i've got less than two weeks to get in shape for a commercial. I look terrible right now. Can you help me . . . please?"

The panic in the model's voice was real. So was the desperation.

Calmly, I responded, "Sure. Meet me at the office at ten o'clock, and we'll formulate a plan."

What I had in this client was someone who had let herself get soft. Extra pounds had piled on, and now remedial work was needed to give her body back its sexy curves, in a very short span of time—less than two weeks. I get calls like hers all the time.

Models, actresses, and others want their legs, buttocks, abs, arms, and other parts of their figures to look as firm and lean as they can be on the set. And why wouldn't they? After all, looking great is their livelihood. Which brings me to you. There's no reason why you can't look picture-perfect, too—and get there rapidly.

How rapidly? Let's just say that if you play your cards right, there could be 5 to 12 pounds less of you in 12 days, with a whole new shape emerging to boot.

I don't blame you if you're skeptical at this point. How can someone get back her gorgeous shape or even reshape her body in 12 days—or, at the very best, see visible changes?

What I will tell you right now is: *This is what I do.*

I get people back in shape fast. I do it for desperate models who have impending assignments. I do it for actors and actresses who must be in top form for upcoming roles. I did it for people on ABC's *Extreme Makeover* who had to be at a healthier weight prior to, or after, having plastic surgery. I do it for guests of my Spa Body Makeover, who come to California to trim down in just a week or two. I do it for clients in my business, Body Makeover Systems, Inc., who want to fast-track their way to shapelier, more defined bodies. This is what I do. And I have been doing it for more than 25 years.

If you give me just 12 days, I'll do it for you, too.

The *12-Day Body Shaping Miracle* is a program of special exercise techniques, coupled with diet, that is designed to alter your body shape so that it gets closer to that ideal of feminine attractiveness: slim waist, streamlined hips and thighs, firm butt, and a lifted bustline. If that's what you want, if that moment has finally come for you, if you're tired of fooling around with exercise programs that don't produce results, then this is the book for you. The program you are about to read will change the shape of your body. You'll learn how to shape and define every area of your body so that you can almost literally sculpt it to achieve a predictable outcome. By *predictable outcome,* I mean the exact way you want your body to look. If you've tried other workout methods in the past but they haven't done the trick, and you have become discouraged in the process, you can now succeed.

The secret: targeted exercise, performed with special movements and employed in a workout that you create and customize for your trouble spots and your unique body type. In addition, you'll be introduced to a totally different approach to cardiovascular exercise that will accelerate your fat loss, but without the drudgery of high-intensity workouts or hours doing cardio. By moving at an acceptable pace and using a special form of breathing—what I call Abdominal Breathing—to oxygenate your body, you'll become trimmer and more fit, plus feel more energetic and invigorated than you have in years. Diet-wise, you'll learn how to recharge your metabolism with food so that you begin to shed fat efficiently, revealing your firm curves.

You'll learn more about these techniques as you and I get further into this book. For now, though, I need something from you: a commitment to unlearn just about everything you've ever been taught about exercise. And I need you to be a willing spirit. Give up your couch time and prepare to become more active. Release what you've been taught or what you've read and be prepared to relearn an entirely new way of exercising. Be open, be willing. Look at it this way: a fresh approach to exercise may be just what you need to get out of a workout or weight-loss rut.

In particular, if you've never done resistance training before, count yourself among the fortunate. You're a blank slate upon which the most effective ways to do it can be written!

Or maybe you have exercised in the past, but without seeing much improvement in your shape. It's one thing to get fit by working out—and that's a great benefit—but exercising without seeing your body become shapelier, trimmer, and younger looking can be a waste of time, like saving money but getting no return on your investment. That's crazy!

Undeniably, the reason you haven't been able to drop those unsightly, unhealthy pounds and resculpt your figure is that you've been exercising incorrectly for your body type. Everyone is built differently; everyone comes in a different size and shape—which is why cookie-cutter or one-workout-fits-all approaches to exercising don't make the grade. How your best friend exercises may work for her but do little for you. By contrast, this program completely customizes your workout to your own body type, trouble spots, and metabolism so that you can see dramatic and rather rapid results.

Through my exclusive Blueprinting system, you'll determine your exact body type. *Body type* refers to your bone structure, your percentage of fat to muscle, your overall proportions, your metabolism, how your body reacts to food. Although every body is different, there are five specific body types, and you're one of them. Knowing your individual type is the first step toward reshaping it to your desired dimensions and following an eating plan geared to your own individual metabolism.

I'll show you the best exercises for your body type and problem areas—exercises that reshape your body fast. If you need to flatten your belly, then I'll show you the single best way to do it. If you need to lift your buns, I'll show you how to have high, rounded glutes like you had when you were younger. If you need great-looking legs, I'll give you exercises that target, tone, and resize your thighs. No, you won't have to do thousands of reps to achieve the shape you want. Working out like that won't give you a tight, toned figure—it will give you a tired body! Once you know your specific body type and understand which exercises work best for you—then do them—you will get to your desired shape quickly.

Before I put another word down on the page, let me say that this is not a fitness book. You can be very fit, yet not even come close to looking the way you want to look or having the body shape you desire. Runners, for example, are very fit, but many are string-bean gaunt, with few appealing curves to their physiques.

So no, this is not a fitness book. This is an art book. You will learn how to look at your body as if it were a piece of raw stone, then visualize the perfect statue you want it to ultimately become. Take in your hand as your chisel and sandpaper my special ways of exercising and dieting and before long, you will have resculpted your body into an aesthetically pleasing new shape. Unlike conventional ways of working out—going to the gym and pumping away on all that equipment for hours at a time—you will discover how to exercise your muscles to shape your body and look exactly the way you want.

Here is the bottom line: How you contract your muscles determines how your muscles look. If you want the long, lean graceful look of a ballet dancer, you can have it. If you want the well-defined, powerful grace of a gymnast, you can have it. If you want the sculpted look of a fitness model, it's yours. How you reshape your body is up to you.

So effective is this approach to body shaping and body sculpting that you can literally see your muscles reshape themselves in a single workout. That kind of near-instant feedback can be so exciting to see, you'll get hooked on this new way of exercising. Every time you use it, you'll be excited about where you can take your body next! You'll have the confidence and the motivation to continue through the initial 12 days and beyond. Once you start on this path, you'll want to keep going. Before long, you will have the toned, curvaceous proportions that can properly fit into a pair of jeans or a skimpy bikini.

But don't take my word for it. Here is what some of my recent clients have posted about their success on the www.provida.com and bodymakeovers.com Web sites.

"My husband and I are winding down Week 1. Already we have both noticed changes in our bodies. I have had those lovely handles on my sides draping over my pant line. Today I woke up, slipped on a pair of jeans, and I couldn't believe my eyes: The love handles are disappearing."

"Even into the 190s, I always had a waist that was very defined and proportionally small, but I'd gotten so fat that it finally went missing. It's back! I caught it reflected in the mirror as I was walking by."

"Cellulite—we all hate it. You know: that cottage cheese look on the behind and legs and wherever. One evening I was looking at my leg while in a short nightgown. My husband looked up from his book and said, 'All the cellulite is gone. Your leg is smooth.' Oh, my gosh! I ran to my full-length mirror and did the close inspection we all do at some time. I was so excited. All visible cellulite was gone."

"Well, I can't believe it. It's been two weeks, and I'm down 22 pounds! I must admit that I was a bit of a skeptic at first but . . . for the first time in my life I think I have hold of something that is going to help me get the weight off, especially in my thighs, which I've been carrying around for a long time, and keep it off."

With this book, I'll teach you, in step-by-step fashion, what these clients have already learned: how to resculpt your trouble areas by selecting specific exercises to tone and shape where you need it. Just as you might remodel your house, this process all starts with a plan to take you where you want to go. This book gives you that plan.

What will happen over the next 12 days will be nothing short of amazing, as long as you stick to the program. You'll learn moves and techniques that will streamline your trouble spots, tighten what needs to be tightened, lift what needs lifting, give your figure symmetry where there was none before, and, in short, transform your shape. Fat will start receding from your body the way the ocean leaves the shore at low tide. Your journey will be challenging, no question, as you learn this truly innovative way of working out and eating.

Why 12 days? So often I have less than two weeks to get clients into shape. Sometimes I have only a week! There's nothing magical about *12,* although it has often been seen as a mystical, or even a lucky, number down through the ages. Whether you believe in luck, pluck, or whatever, though, this 12-day program works. It is based on scientific principles of exercise more than anything else, plus more than 25 years of my own experience doing physique makeovers. It is a simple solution to the perfect-body equation.

Please understand: When I designed this as a 12-day program, I did not intend it as a gimmick. Gimmicks don't work. They never do; they never will. What I'm introducing you to is meant to be the beginning of a better, more efficient way to exercise—a method that can surely change your shape very rapidly, and if you continue to use it, you can develop the sexiest, most beautiful body you've ever had. Twelve days is what it will take to show you that this is the best way for you to exercise to change your shape. By the end of 12 days, you'll see flattering and remarkable improvements in the way you look and feel. So flattering and remarkable, in fact, that you'll be motivated to make this method a way of life.

For you to get the body you want, you must approach this program as a priority assignment, with your total focus on achieving the shape you desire. That means you must concentrate, a day at a time, on following the diet and exercise instructions given in this book, without deviating from them. This is something that is simple and something that is doable.

What happens after the initial 12 days is that you're on your way to establishing a new exercise habit! The 12 days get you started, and once they're over you'll be able to see a change in your body. If you do this program correctly, if you learn how to contract (flex) your muscles, if you follow the cardio portion of the program, if you do your diet, if you rest your body, this program will set you on the path toward being sculpted and streamlined, with your exact desired specifications taking form. You'll emerge stronger and more self-assured.

How to Use This Book

What I've just described is exactly what can happen to you when you start working out according to your body type, using moves designed to correct and streamline your trouble areas while staying true to my dietary principles of balanced, metabolism-boosting nutrition. You can also chisel away those soft spots and replace them with shapely curves.

I have organized this book around two major parts. Within each part are chapters that cover the specifics of this plan. It is best if you read through the entire book first to get familiar with the plan and what you'll be doing. Then go back, chapter by chapter, and put into action each part of the plan. One of the first actions you'll take, for example, is to blueprint your body (chapter 2) so that you'll know which body type you have. Then you can customize your diet and exercise program to that body type. Next you'll want to get into the proper attitude in order to motivate yourself mentally for success and think like a makeover winner (this is covered in chapter 3).

Part 2 covers the exercise techniques and principles on which the *12-Day Body Shaping Miracle* is based. These are specifically designed to reshape your body, burn body fat, and build shapely muscle in all the right places. You'll learn which exercises to do for your shape and how to exercise correctly for more rapid results. Your diet is critical to success, so make sure you follow the nutrition plan for your body type. This information is outlined in detail in chapter 8.

I have also included three appendices. Pay particular attention to appendix A, which covers exercise and nutrition exceptions if you have any special medical conditions, such as diabetes or high blood pressure.

Like so many of my makeover clients, with these techniques and this plan, you'll ultimately be able to show off your sexy curves and great new body.

Are you ready for a transformation? If so, give me 12 days, and you, too, will start to see a lean, sexy body that you'll love.

1

Slimming and Shaping Your Body

CHAPTER 1

The Shape of Things to Come

Look around you someday—at the mall, in your workplace, at social events, in the gym. You'll observe that everyone comes in a wide variety of sizes and shapes. Every person on this planet is unique—including you. That's why, if you want to change your shape, you must have a program that is precisely tailored to you. One-size-fits-all plans simply do not work for changing your body shape, because one size does not fit all when it comes to exercise and nutrition.

Just keep in mind that each body requires a different workout, and a different diet. You achieve the shape you want by following the correct workout—one that targets trouble spots and matches your body type—along with a diet that supports your unique metabolic needs. Let's dig into this strategy a little deeper, and you'll be encouraged by the amount of power you have to radically change your shape. Here's a clue: There's a lot more to it than what you were born with (otherwise known as genetics).

Because most body types are inherited and genes don't change, we were all born with a basic shape that stays genetically fixed. But genes don't sentence you to an unappealing figure. You can remodel your entire body with a diet and an exercise program customized for your individual body type. Diet and cardiovascular exercise, for example, transform your body by getting rid of unwanted excess fat, by speeding up your metabolism, and by preventing the tendency for your body to gain excess fat as you get older. This program does the trick by coaxing your body into burning a higher percentage of fat than it normally would through

3

diet alone. The higher the percentage of body fat you burn, and the more you challenge your muscles through my special brand of exercising, the faster your results, and the faster your desired shape will emerge.

You will learn to look at your figure very critically, then decide exactly what body parts you want to change and reshape. You will select exercises that accomplish this and systematically put them into a workout routine that is uniquely yours, and no one else's. Your exercise equipment needs are few. Exercise that uses weights or bands or some other form of resistance that challenges your muscles grants you the power to build up or scale down specific areas of your body, giving it more shapely, proportional contours. Thus, you can change your body type to a degree as long as you employ the right mixture of diet and exercise.

What Factors Affect Your Shape?

The shape you're in today is determined by three primary factors: your skeleton, your muscle, and your body fat. Your skeleton, or bone structure, is a frame upon which the other two factors are draped. It's the only aspect of your shape that you generally cannot change. Of course, if you do no exercise at all, that bone structure will begin to degrade through lack of use, and osteoporosis, a bone-thinning disease, can set in. I suppose if you did no exercise at all, you could change your bone structure negatively by default through a detrimental, wasting-away process. Bones do need resistance, in the form of exercise, to maintain their integrity and stay strong well into your golden years. By placing some stress on your bone structure, resistance training helps protect your bones by stimulating them to produce new cells. This process helps protect you against osteoporosis.

Muscle, which moves the 206 bones in your body, gives your figure its most desirable shape and its sexy curves. Firm muscles are attractive and serve to lift other types of tissue that might otherwise sag. You have enormous control over the shape, the size, and the symmetry of your muscles. By *symmetry*, I am referring to the relationship or balance among muscle groups as they line up on your body. A good example of a symmetrical body for a woman is a trim hourglass figure.

Unfortunately, as muscles age, they lose cells—and along with that loss comes a corresponding loss in firmness and body shape. Existing muscle cells shrink and become less contractile and less flexible, all of which makes them more susceptible to strains and pulls. The good news is, however, that even aging muscles can become reconditioned. Virtually all it takes is resistance training, done consistently and properly, and your muscles can become younger looking again—and with them, your body.

Just as your muscles form the desirable part of your shape, body fat tends to contribute to an undesirable shape. One exception to this would be your breasts. These are composed of fatty tissue and give the female form a desirable shape—unless, of course, they sag or are out of proportion with the rest of your figure. Special exercises and techniques, however, can lift your breasts, strengthening and firming the surrounding tissue, and thus giving the illusion of a sexier bustline. You'll learn about, and apply, these methods here.

As a woman, you tend to gain weight more easily than a man would, and you often have to work harder to get it off. A major reason for this is that women have more fat-storing enzymes in their bodies, while men have more fat-releasing enzymes. (*Enzymes* are catalysts in the body that mediate or speed up various physiological reactions.) With more fat-storing enzymes, fat cells tend to enlarge, creating unsightly body fat that mars a woman's natural, sexy shape. Here is a piece of encouraging news: Cardio exercise increases fat-releasing enzymes—which is why walking, jogging, running, and other forms of cardio are so effective at burning fat.

Hormones and Body Fat

The accumulation of body fat and its redistribution are also related to aging. On average, an older body is a flabbier body. You've probably noticed, too, that excess fat settles in different places at different stages in your life. When you're a teenager or young adult, fat is fairly evenly distributed throughout your body, and it's held rather tightly in place, without the sagging brought on by aging. By the time you're 30 or 40, though, it heads straight to your hips, buttocks, and thighs. The female hormone estrogen, which activates and multiplies fat-storing enzymes, directs this shifting pattern of fat accumulation.

For women, a sudden increase in weight often occurs following menopause, with fat collecting mostly around the waist, as well as on the hips and thighs. Not only does this raise obesity-related health concerns, but the weight gain can also be emotionally troubling for aging women.

In a research study conducted at Oregon Health & Science University, scientists observed a group of 46 pre- and postmenopausal women. In the postmenopausal group, some of the women involved in the study were receiving hormone replacement therapy; others were not. By analyzing data from study participants, researchers determined that the drop in estrogen levels commonly associated with menopause is linked to an increase in a form of the hormone cortisol, which has been implicated in the formation of excess abdominal fat. Another key finding was that postmenopausal women who were not receiving hormone replacement therapy had higher cortisol levels than those who were receiving therapy. On average, these untreated women with higher cortisol levels also witnessed an increase in abdominal fat when compared with women receiving the therapy. These findings also suggest that estrogen replacement therapy protects women from developing high cortisol levels and increased abdominal fat.

Because it appears that estrogen replacement therapy can help protect you from increased abdominal fat, I frequently recommend that women have their hormone levels tested by their physician and look into replacement therapy with bio-identical hormones—estrogen or progesterone or both—taken under a doctor's supervision. Extracted from soy or yams, bio-identical hormones are similar to the hormones estrogen and progesterone that your body makes naturally. As such, when they enter the bloodstream, they interact with your cells in the same way that your own hormones do. If bio-identical hormones are a therapy you might want to consider, please consult with your physician as you would on all medical issues.

Whether or not you elect to explore treatment with bio-identical hormones with your doctor, resistance training helps keep these aging- and hormone-related changes in fat distribution to a minimum. Much of what we consider aging—the accumulation of body fat, the loss of strength and bone density, and the decrease in flexibility—is actually due to inactivity.

What You Can Do About Your Shape

With the exception of your bone structure, you can change your shape by sculpting your muscles and losing body fat. The methods and the program that I recommend in this book are among the very best ways to accomplish that. The resistance-training techniques and the exercises you'll learn in upcoming chapters will help transform your figure in ways you never thought possible—better proportions, less body fat, greater muscle tone and development, and more. Not only will you get curvier muscles, but you'll also rid your body of unwanted fat by developing lean muscle. Firm, strong muscles are metabolically active. This means they can burn body fat more efficiently than can untoned muscle, even at rest.

By including my cardio recommendations, you can more than double your fat-burning power. In fact, one study found that people who combined resistance-training exercises with aerobics lost two and a half times more body fat than those who performed cardio only! The nutrition guidelines you'll follow will further stimulate fat burning.

Before moving on, there's one critical issue affecting your body type that I must address if you want to get the body you desire.

Stop This Bad Habit and Start Changing Your Shape Today

Do you smoke cigarettes? If so, your smoking habit is making your body store fat around your waist and upper torso. That's the conclusion of a growing and compelling amount of research into the relationship between fat distribution and smoking. One large-scale study, in particular, analyzed data from 21,828 men and women who were 45 to 79 years of age and found that the smokers tended to be chubby around the waist. In another study of nearly 12,000 pre- and post-menopausal women aged 40 to 73, the women's waistline increased as the number of cigarettes smoked per day increased. What's the connection? By unbalancing your endocrine system (glands that secrete hormones), smoking affects fat distribution by causing fat to be stored centrally—around the middle.

Of course, these changes to your waistline don't have to be permanent. Other research has found that if you stop smoking, less fat will collect around your waist. So is smoking cessation a way to influence and control your body shape? I'd say so!

What to Expect

If you review this discussion of factors influencing your body shape, it's obvious that you have a great deal of control over your figure and how it ultimately looks. That's incredibly powerful news, because you have the power to change your shape to your exact specifications through proper exercise, diet, and other lifestyle alterations.

The advantages of following the *12-Day Body Shaping Miracle* are that, number one, my exercise methods are designed to focus on critical areas of your figure to get them in shape, and number two, the customized diet you will follow is designed to burn fat from your entire body.

As you follow the guidelines in this book, you will be redesigning the total package of your body. That's what this approach does—adds a bit here, takes some away there, and before long, a more balanced shape emerges. No body parts are overdeveloped or underdeveloped at the expense of others. You will remodel your figure with a diet and exercise program geared for your goals.

Thus, this program can transform your figure in ways you never thought possible—better proportions, less body fat, greater muscle tone and development, and more. It's all about maximizing your unique shape and looking fabulous in your clothes.

As you go forward on this program, expect to experience at least 11 great benefits:

- Slenderized, firm thighs
- Trimmer hips
- Flatter abdominals
- Better symmetry
- Loss of inches in the right places
- Steady, satisfying weight loss
- Improved fitness
- Ample energy
- Greater self-confidence
- Positive feelings about yourself and your body
- Overall sense of well-being

As long as you stick to the diet and exercise guidelines in this book, you can achieve all these wonderful results. A new body can be yours!

CHAPTER 2

Blueprint Your Body

Changing your shape begins on paper, first with a written question-naire and corresponding illustrations that together pinpoint your body type accu-rately and easily. I'm referring to my Body Type Blueprinting system, which I'll explain in this chapter. This Blueprint will help you determine which of five stan-dard body types, or shapes, you have; you can then individualize your exercise pro-gram and your diet. By completing the questionnaire, you'll identify your body type and be on your way to customizing a plan that works for you. So grab a pen or pencil, and let's get started.

Blueprinting Questionnaire: What Body Type Are You?

Body typing is a way to describe the percentage of fat to muscle on your frame, your bone structure, your overall proportions, and your metabolism, since there can be a correlation between body type and how efficiently your body metabolizes food for fuel. There are five different body types, each based on solid science, and one of them will fit you. This questionnaire is a very easy method for identifying your body type. It takes approximately 5 to 10 minutes to answer all 48 questions and complete the scoring. Read each statement carefully and circle only those statements that best describe you right now. Be as honest as you can; there are no right or wrong answers. Take your time and do not rush through this questionnaire.

Once you're finished with the questionnaire, you'll know which of five body types you have. Then you'll be ready to move directly into the next chapters, where you'll learn which exercises and diet are right for you. That means you'll be able to start changing your shape, losing weight, and looking better than you have in a long time—right away.

Check the box beside each comment that most accurately describes you. Remember, be honest in your answers.

- ❏ 1. When I gain weight, it's all over my entire body.
- ❏ 2. I have always been athletic, but recently the pounds have begun to creep up.
- ❏ 3. There was a time, after I graduated from high school, when I could eat practically anything I wanted and never gain an ounce.
- ❏ 4. It seems like no matter how little I eat, I gain weight.
- ❏ 5. For as long as I can remember, all I had to do was look at food and I would gain weight.
- ❏ 6. If I am even an hour late for a regular meal, I get ravenously hungry.
- ❏ 7. Even if I lost all the fat I wanted, I'd never be a skinny model type. I have more meat on my bones than that.
- ❏ 8. I have lots of energy. People are always amazed at how much I get done in a day.
- ❏ 9. Most of the time I can hide my weight in my clothes, but I wouldn't consider being seen in a swimsuit.
- ❏ 10. I am rarely hungry at mealtimes.
- ❏ 11. Obesity runs in my family; many close members of my family are 50 pounds or more overweight.
- ❏ 12. I get hungry very soon after I eat.
- ❏ 13. If all the fat on my body disappeared, I think that I'd look great.
- ❏ 14. If all the fat on my body disappeared, I might be skinny or bony.
- ❏ 15. To get my ideal body, I will have to lose one to two dress sizes (say, from size 8 to 6 or 4).

16. To get my ideal body, I will have to lose three to four dress sizes (say, from size 14 to 8 or 6).

17. To get my ideal body, I will have to lose five or more dress sizes (say, from size 18 to 8 or 6).

18. If I go more than two or three hours without eating, I get shaky or irritable.

19. There are parts of my body that are too muscular—my butt or thighs or arms.

20. At the same time that I lose weight, I would like to increase the size of some of my muscles to give my body shape and definition.

21. It is only as I got older or had children that I started to have trouble with my weight.

22. I have very low energy levels much of the time.

23. I worry that I'm so overweight, it's jeopardizing my health.

24. If I go a long time without eating, I get a feeling of panic.

25. As far as I can remember, I have never been so thin that people would call me bony or skinny.

26. Parts of my body are too thin—skinny arms, thighs, or calves.

27. When I get more physical activity in my life, my body loses fat fairly quickly.

28. I need to lose weight all over my body.

29. Because of my weight, it's very hard for me to do any kind of exercise.

30. If I don't eat on schedule, I simply can't control what I eat at the next meal.

31. Even though I may have more fat than I want, the body underneath is still pretty solid; it's hard or firm when I flex my muscles.

32. At some point in my adult life, people have said to me, "You should gain weight; you look too thin."

33. There are parts of my body that are *not* overweight.

34. I currently eat only twice a day.

35. I have had serious weight problems for nearly my entire life.

36. Sometimes when I get up too quickly, I feel light-headed or dizzy.

37. If I had to describe myself as either strong or weak physically, I would tend to say strong.

38. If I had to describe myself as either strong or weak physically, I would tend to say weak.

39. I tend to gain weight in specific areas (belly, love handles, thighs) while much of the rest of my body stays normal.

40. I have been off and on diets for much of my adult life.

41. I believe that I am genetically doomed to be fat and will always be fat.

42. After exercise, I often feel like I'm starving.

43. If I flex my arm, I can feel a muscle.

44. More than being overweight, my problem is that my body lacks shape or definition.

45. I have only had trouble with my weight for the last three to five years.

46. I used to be very athletic, but I don't even recognize my body anymore.

47. If I had to pick a shape to describe my body, it would probably be round.

48. If I'm tense or anxious, eating a candy bar, bread, or pasta tends to calm me down.

Scoring and Interpretation

Next, follow these steps to total your answers and identify your unique body type.

STEP 1 Circle the number below of each corresponding question you checked in the questionnaire. For example, if you checked number #11 in the questionnaire, you would circle number #11 in column 5.

1	2	3	4	5	6
1	2	3	4	5	6
7	8	9	10	11	12
13	14	15	16	17	18
19	20	21	22	23	24
25	26	27	28	29	30
31	32	33	34	35	36
37	38	39	40	41	42
43	44	45	46	47	48

Total the number of circles in each column.

STEP 2 In the chart above, count the number of circles in each column and write the total in the spaces at the bottom of the columns. *If you have five or more circles in column 5, you are a Body Type A. If you are not a Body Type A, please continue.*

STEP 3 Look at column 1 and column 2 and determine which of those two columns has the most circles. That *column number* (1 or 2) is your *primary number*. For example, if the total of column 1 is 3 and the total of column 2 is 5, then your primary number is 2. Write your primary number in the box below.

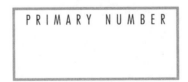

PRIMARY NUMBER

Note: If you have the same number in columns 1 and 2, your primary number is 1.

STEP 4

Look at column 3 and column 4 and determine which of those two columns has the most circles. That column number is your *secondary number*. Write that number in the box below.

```
SECONDARY NUMBER


```

Note: If you have the same number in columns 3 and 4, your secondary number is 4.

STEP 5

Use your primary number and your secondary number to identify your body type:

- If your *primary number* is *1* and your *secondary number* is *4*, your *body type* is B.
- If your *primary number* is *1* and your *secondary number* is *3*, your *body type* is C.
- If your *primary number* is *2* and your *secondary number* is *4*, your *body type* is D.
- If your *primary number* is *2* and your *secondary number* is *3*, your *body type* is E.

Write your body type in the box below.

```
MY BODY TYPE


```

IMPORTANT NOTE: All readers should consult with their physician before beginning this, or any, diet and exercise program. Special consideration should be taken by you and your doctor if you have more than two circles in column 6. You may have a tendency toward low blood sugar, technically known as hypoglycemia. Please read the section on hypoglycemia in appendix A, Workout and Diet Customizations for Special Medical Conditions. If you had five or more checks in column 6, you may be very hypoglycemic, and you should discuss this condition with your physician before you begin the *12-Day Body Shaping Miracle*.

In addition, if you checked statement 36, you may have low blood pressure. Please read the information on low blood pressure in appendix A and consult with your physician before beginning the program.

Understanding Your Body Type

Now that you've identified your body type, read this section carefully. I list for you the major body composition and metabolic characteristics that correspond to your body type, along with general body-shaping objectives to consider. In parentheses are the technical descriptions of each body type: *endomorph, endo-meso, meso-endo, endo-ecto,* and *ecto-endo.* These descriptions are based on a well-known and medically approved system, developed in the 1940s by a man named Dr. William H. Sheldon, that classifies people by body types. By photographing and measuring 46,000 men and women, Sheldon and his colleagues eventually developed 88 distinct categories. To simplify his system, he then created the three major divisions of ectomorph (a thin shape with little muscle), endomorph (a round, soft shape), and mesomorph (muscular and athletic). Within each of these major divisions are "degrees of dominance." Although some people are purely endomorph, mesomorph, or ectomorph, most of us are a mixture of body types with one type being dominant. An endo-meso, for example, is someone who has the characteristics of an endomorph (tends to gain fat easily) but also has quite a bit of lean muscle on her body. An ecto-endo is like the ectomorph (thin with small bones and joints) but puts on weight as easily as an endomorph.

Regardless of your individual body type, you have the physical potential to develop a beautiful body and an attractive shape through diet and exercise. Knowing your body type is the first step toward attaining those goals.

Each of the following descriptions is accompanied by an illustration of that particular body type. These are generic sketches to further help you determine your shape. Don't expect to see an exact match of your body, however. Simply look to see if one of the drawings looks similar to you in terms of where your body gains weight.

Body Type A (Endomorph)

Your body is nearly 100 percent endomorph, with a higher-than-desirable percentage of body fat distributed at and below the waist. You have probably always had trouble managing your weight and tend to be quite heavy. You put on weight easily, and for the most part you gain it evenly over your entire body. This gives you a softer, rounder physique, with a tendency toward obesity. Other identifying characteristics include:

Body Shape Characteristics
- Your physique may be shaped much like a *circle*—large and round.
- You may be larger around your waist or in your hip and buttocks regions, or even all over your entire body.
- You have more body fat on your frame relative to lean muscle.
- Your muscles are underdeveloped.
- Your body is soft, and your flesh is loose.
- You may have been overweight as a child.

Metabolic Characteristics
- Yours is the slowest metabolism of all five body types.
- You have a tendency to metabolize any food taken into your body as body fat.
- You have a ready disposition toward gaining body fat.
- It may be difficult for you to lose body fat.

Body-Shaping Objectives
- Stick to the eating plan for your body type.
- Overcome a sluggish metabolism to burn more fat.
- Create more lean muscle on your body to increase your metabolism and burn fat.
- Do enough cardio to start shedding the fat that's concealing your shape.
- Shrink, tighten, and flatten your abs to reduce centrally deposited body fat.
- Tighten, minimize, and firm your lower body, with possible extra attention to your butt, and inner and outer thighs.
- Balance your figure by working your upper body to be in proportion with your lower body.

Body Type B (Endo-Meso)

Your dominant body type is endomorph, but with the solid muscular development of a mesomorph. You tend to be thick all over, with loose flesh over the muscle. What's more, you gain weight easily and may be significantly (20 or more pounds) overweight. Other identifying characteristics include:

Body Shape Characteristics
- You may be shaped like a *triangle,* with body fat concentrated in your hips, thighs, and buttocks. In addition, you may also have thick arms. (Typically, endo-mesos are thick throughout their bodies.)
- You may have narrow shoulders, a small chest, and an average waistline.
- You have strong muscle tone beneath your layer of body fat.

Metabolic Characteristics
- You gain fat easily.
- You have trouble losing weight.
- Your metabolism is sluggish.
- You build and maintain muscle easily.

Body-Shaping Objectives
- Stick to the eating plan for your body type.
- Overcome a sluggish metabolism to burn more fat.
- Build up your upper body to create more proportion relative to your lower body, especially if your shoulders tend to slope or you want to create more of a V-shape in your back to give the illusion of a smaller waistline.
- Create a little more lean muscle on your body to increase your metabolism and burn fat.
- Do enough cardio to start shedding the fat that's concealing your shape.
- Tighten, minimize, and firm your lower body, with possible extra attention to your butt and thighs.

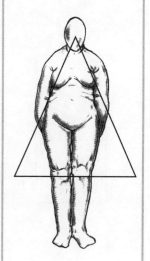

Body Type C (Meso-Endo)

You have a strong, muscular body—the kind you might see on athletes. In other words, the mesomorph characteristics are dominant. Yet like an endomorph, you have a difficult time reducing body fat. Oversized muscles are almost as big a problem as having too much body fat. Other identifying characteristics include:

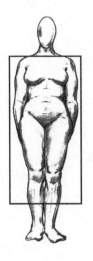

Body Composition Characteristics
- Your frame is generally thick-bodied. Shape-wise, it may resemble a *rectangle*, roughly the same width at the shoulders, waist, and hips.
- There is a covering of fat over your muscle. (This fat might be intramuscular, like the marbling in red meat.)
- Your body has tight, hard flesh, with fatty tissue covering it.
- You may have broad shoulders.

Metabolic Characteristics
- You gain body fat fairly easily.
- Your metabolism isn't as sluggish as other body types because of your muscular development.
- You build and maintain muscle tissue very easily.

Body-Shaping Objectives
- Stick to the eating plan for your body type.
- Do enough cardio to start shedding the fat that's concealing your shape.
- Trim fat off your body (with cardio) and tone your abdominal muscles back into shape using short-range abdominal exercises.
- In your resistance training, focus on more repetitions with lighter resistances to slenderize your already muscular figure.

Body Type D (Endo-Ecto)

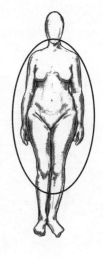

You may be significantly overweight and inclined to gain weight easily—like an endomorph. Yet you have the slight frame of an ectomorph. You have very little muscle on your body, and your flesh tends to look loose and flabby. Other identifying characteristics include:

Body Shape Characteristics
- Your shape may resemble an *oval*, with a fuller chest, no apparent waistline, and narrow shoulders and legs.
- Your weight may tend to congregate around your waist.
- You may have a skinny body underneath the body fat, with very little muscle tissue.
- You may have a slight frame, and you're generally small-boned, but over time you've rounded out with a greater percentage of body fat, particularly on your arms, legs, and hips.

Metabolic Characteristics
- Your metabolism is somewhat more sluggish than other body types.
- You tend to gain weight easily.
- You struggle to build and maintain lean muscle.

Body-Shaping Objectives
- Stick to the eating plan for your body type.
- Create a slimmer waistline through short-range abdominal work and cardio.
- Work toward better proportion by changing your oval shape into more of an hourglass figure. Your resistance training should focus on fewer repetitions, and heavier resistances, to build your upper body and tone your lower body.

Body Type E (Ecto-Endo)

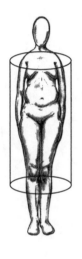

You're essentially a lanky, thin person (like an ectomorph), but you've gained too much weight in places. Your weight problems may be relatively new; at one time, you might have found it hard to put on weight. You have very little muscle tissue, and you may actually be skinny or bony on parts of your body, while other parts—your abdomen, waist, or thighs—tend to be overweight with loose, droopy flesh. Other identifying characteristics include:

Body Shape Characteristics

- Where once your body may have been described as a stick, with a thin, lean look, now you've rounded out, filling out in places, and your physique resembles a *tube.* In other words, there is a skinny, bony frame underneath areas of body fat.
- You have very little muscle tissue.
- You may have skinny arms or legs that are covered with a layer of body fat.

Metabolic Characteristics

- Your overall metabolic rate isn't as slow as other body types, but it's still not fast enough to keep you lean.
- It's difficult for you to burn enough calories to keep from gaining weight.
- You have trouble building and maintaining lean muscle.
- At a younger age, you could eat anything you wanted without ever gaining weight.

Body-Shaping Objectives

- Stick to the eating plan for your body type.
- Create more lean muscle on your body to increase your metabolism and keep fat from accumulating.
- Add curves to your upper and lower body with resistance training that focuses on fewer repetitions coupled with heavier resistances. This will help put some extra dimension in your figure and help develop lean muscle. If you have never done resistance training before, however, you will want to start with lighter resistances and build slowly and gradually to heavier resistances.

Changing Your Shape

Once you've identified your correct body type using the Blueprinting Questionnaire, you're ready to start changing your shape. With the information you've gathered here, you're equipped with the first, and perhaps the most important, piece of the body-shaping puzzle we're putting together. Hold on to this information, because it will help you put your workout plan into action. From there, reshaping your body to your exact specifications is a result of losing fat, firming up, and proportionalizing muscle. That is exactly what this program will do for you.

CHAPTER 3

Master the Mind–Body Connection

The actual doing of the program on the *12-Day Body Shaping Miracle* is fairly straightforward: You shape, tone, and define your muscles by following the workout methods and exercises I will give you in this book. And you enhance your progress with wise, customized nutritional choices, as outlined in chapter 8. But truth be told, the success of this program doesn't start with the body-shaping methods or the nutrition principles you'll follow. It starts in your head—with some important mind–body skills. The sooner you apply those skills, the faster you'll make progress and push your entire body-shaping effort to new levels.

In this chapter, I'll give you several mind–body skills that can make this program more effective, more fun, and even easier. These skills will become a tool for enormous progress when they're used daily and can lead to personal transformation. Make a commitment to use them not only during the next 12 days, but beyond, and they'll become stepping-stones to a fitter, trimmer, and shapelier body.

Skill 1. Visualization

When I started changing my own body (and developing the foundation for the techniques that would later become my makeover programs), I used to fantasize about how I wanted to look—chiseled abs, large biceps, muscular shoulders, a V-shaped back—the whole package. I wasn't just wishing I had an in-shape physique; I was very specific about what I wanted to accomplish.

I'd start by finding images of the body I wanted. I'd study those images in detail. Then I'd imagine the fat melting off my body, and my individual muscles changing shape in very specific ways. This process of mental concentration—which I called daydreaming—helped me stay focused on my goal and eventually played a huge part in helping me get exactly the body I wanted for bodybuilding competitions. Then one day, I looked in the mirror, and there it was: I could see the physique I'd envisioned for myself begin to emerge. It was very exciting. Seeing yourself change is a very empowering experience.

Without knowing it, I was utilizing a technique that is widely known today as visualization. This is the process of creating a mental picture of achievement. You form in your mind what you want your new shape to look like. While this may still seem like daydreaming, in fact visualization is now accepted in a variety of disciplines to help people achieve fantastic goals. Visualization is what helps Olympic athletes and professional ballplayers perform at their personal best. It is what has helped many cancer patients overcome life-threatening illness. And it is what will allow you to achieve just about any goal you set for yourself.

The conception of an event, or an end point, in your mind is the beginning of its existence, and without a clear image of what the outcome will be, the manifestation of that event is almost impossible. In other words, if you don't know what you want and don't believe you can get it, you can't. However, if you have a clear picture of what you want to accomplish and the solid belief that you can make it happen, then success is almost guaranteed—provided you formulate a realistic plan and diligently follow it.

Trust me, if you use your mind to envision what you can be, you will begin to make the right choices, the healthy choices, to become what you see in your mind's eye. Your mind is a very powerful force that can help you achieve your inner vision of your desired outer appearance. The body you see yourself achieving, no matter how misshapen you feel now, is ultimately the body you want and will have.

Here's how you can start to practice visualization: Get in a comfortable position, sitting or lying with your eyes closed. In your mind's eye, picture your body the exact way you want it to be shaped. With as much detail as possible, think proportion. Think lean defined muscles everywhere on your body. Think about how you will look and feel physically and emotionally when you have the body of your dreams. Take it a step further. See yourself looking sexy and fabulous in a swimsuit or other revealing outfit. Picture yourself out in public wearing new, formfitting clothes and how great you'll look in them. Dream away!

Make this scene as vivid as possible, using as many of your senses as you can. The more senses you call to mind in your visualization, the greater the impact of the image. Notice how you look, what you can hear, smell, feel, and taste. Notice your surroundings, whether there are other people around, and anything else that is part of your success scenario. Notice how good it feels to be in those clothes and in your new body. The more vivid you can make the new you in your mind, the more successful you will be.

The vision you have for your future body is what you will achieve with your individualized workouts, diet, and rest. If you have a clear vision of where you want to go, it makes it easier to get there. Visualization is absolutely vital because it actually encourages your body to follow your brain's plan, and this mind–body link enhances your ability to change your shape and lose body fat.

Do something else with me, too. When you eat your prescribed meals on this program, visualize the food's nutrients going directly to your muscles. Think about the protein making your muscles firmer and better defined and the carbohydrates fueling your body for greater energy. Not only does visualization add an inspiring dimension to your workout, but it may also give you a new attitude toward eating healthier foods.

Do your visualization exercise at least once a day for about 10 minutes. Keep the image of your new body in the forefront of your mind. You can also use visualization when you feel yourself giving into a craving, or when you're experiencing stress. You'll find that this exercise is a terrific way to rid your body and your mind of all kinds of burdens.

Skill 2. Mantras

Accompany your visualizations by what's known as a *mantra*—a personal statement that is meaningful to you, and positive. Mantras are really a form of self-talk, the dialogue you have with yourself in your mind. The function of the mantra is to give you direction, as well as to ignite your enthusiasm and motivation.

You might tell yourself: *I intend to create a lean, sculpted, sexy body . . . I'm going to lose weight and fit into a smaller size . . . I'm going to look fabulous in my outfit . . . People are going to enjoy seeing me succeed . . . I love my body, and I'll love it more when I lose those pounds.* Direct your thoughts and concentration to what is affirming, what is positive. Creating an unshakable positive attitude is critical to your achievement on this program, and your self-talk, or mantra, will help you have one.

Not only will your mantra help you focus on doing this program successfully, but it will also silence the negative self-talk that all of us hear in our heads once in a while: *I'm too tired to exercise today* or *I feel like slipping off my diet just this once.* If you find this kind of unproductive self-talk seeping into your mind, immediately switch to your mantras, and you'll cancel out the negative inner dialogue. At the same time, listen to your body. If you really are too tired to exercise, then your body may need rest.

Skill 3. Mini-Goals

As you go through this program, I recommend that you stay focused on what specifically you want to achieve each day. This will make it easier to wake up in the morning and get going. In other words, set mini-goals daily. Sticking to anything for a single day is a cinch. You don't have to think about doing the program for 12 days. Instead you concentrate on *today*. When you take it a day at a time, it becomes incredibly easy. A mini-goal can be anything that helps you stay focused on what you want to achieve in a single day of the program:

- *Today I will do my body-shaping workout and give it my all.*
- *Today I will practice my visualizations.*

- *Today I will stick to my eating plan 100 percent.*
- *Today I will do my cardio exercise.*
- *Today I will drink the recommended amount of water.*

Whatever your mini-goals are, I suggest that you write them down and post them where you can see them. Recording your mini-goals on paper or in your computer drives home the need for doing them. Make sure your mini-goals are clear and specific, too. Without this kind of clarity, it is difficult to concentrate on your actions and avoid distractions.

Skill 4. Exercise Concentration

One of the single most important aspects of reshaping your body is to really concentrate on the muscles you're working. Too often, we focus on getting from exercise to exercise or completing a specific number of sets and repetitions—in other words, just getting through the workout. Or we let our minds wander to our love life, what's for dinner, the blaring television, or other distractions that can only hinder performance. You need to block these all out and get inside your muscles.

One of the keys to this level of concentration is to slow down each repetition of the exercise; do not rush through the moves. In a controlled fashion, slowly move the resistance so that you feel yourself really working the muscle, instead of just trying to finish the set. Resist the temptation to let momentum take over the exercise movement, and stay focused on the muscle you're working. (In chapter 6, I'll give you exact guidelines on how to locate the targeted muscle or muscle groups with each exercise so that you understand where to focus.)

What I want you to do with each exercise is concentrate on, and feel, the targeted muscle or muscle groups you're working. Once you're able to focus on the body part you're exercising, each repetition suddenly becomes more productive. Also, be sure that you contract, or flex, the muscles you're working. You want to feel the muscle contract from the beginning of the movement through to the end. Shaping the muscle is about isolating it, squeezing it, and exerting full control over every inch of the movement. In many cases, you'll want to hold the contraction for a certain number of seconds. Through doing this every time you exercise, you will always be able to feel every muscle you're working.

Achieving this kind of concentration doesn't come naturally. It requires practice. But there is an important dividend: With the ability to get inside your muscles during your workout, you'll be able to concentrate fully and remain resistant to potential distractions.

Listen to your body during every workout. Tune in to the feedback that your mind and body provide during exercise, such as: Can you see changes in your shape? Are you getting stronger? Do you have more endurance? Staying aware of your progress during your workout keeps you connected to what your body is doing and how it is feeling.

Skill 5. De-Stressing

When it comes to getting in shape, one of the most fascinating mind–body links has to do with stress. A medical definition of *stress* is "something that disturbs a person's mental and physical well-being." A more common definition is that stress is a heightened emotional response to both everyday and out-of-the-ordinary circumstances.

However you define it, stress that goes unresolved contributes to one figure problem you don't want: a bulging belly. Why? Fat in the abdominal area functions differently from fat elsewhere in the body. It contains a greater blood supply, as well as more cellular receptors for cortisol, a stress hormone. (Receptors function like door locks situated on cell walls: They let hormones and nutrients into cells.) Cortisol levels rise and fall throughout the day, but when you are under chronic stress, the amount of the hormone your body produces remains elevated. Cortisol, in particular, isn't metabolized well. With a lot of stress and, consequently, high cortisol levels, more fat is dumped in the abdominal area since there are more cortisol receptors there. Fat cells in your abdominal region are very sensitive to cortisol, and they tend to grow in size when they hook up with this hormone.

In fact, research shows that people who are depressed, suffering from anxiety, out of a job, or recently divorced—all stress-related difficulties—have too much fat distributed around their waists. This type of fat has often been called "stress fat" because it is caused by high levels of stress-induced cortisol.

When researchers at the University of California–San Francisco put 59 premenopausal women through stress tests in a laboratory, they discovered that those who had greater abdominal fat performed worse on the tests and secreted significantly more cortisol than those without fat tummies. This study and others point out that greater life stress contributes to greater fat distribution around the waist, and cortisol is the hormonal culprit.

If your belly bulge won't budge, even if you're faithful to your diet, you need to add a stress-reduction program to your daily routine. This might involve putting more balance in your life, so that you have time for pleasure, relaxation, and spiritual fulfillment—all life choices that will counteract the negative effects of stress. Or it might involve a program to change your thinking. In truth, it's not really people or events that stress you out but your reactions to, and interpretations of, those stressors. If you can reframe or mentally reinterpret the stressors in your life, you'll be less stressed by what happens around you.

Sometimes resolving chronic stress may require more serious measures—like seeing a counselor. He or she may help you identify strategies to cope with and ultimately resolve the underlying issues perpetuating the distress. Or you may want to pour out your heart to a friend. Just talking to someone you trust can make you feel much better.

One way you can instantly reduce stress is through breathing. When your body perceives a stressful situation, breathing becomes shallow and your heart rate increases. Your upper back and neck muscles become tight. Taking slow, deep breaths, as recommended in my Abdominal Breathing method, can calm your body and mind in less than a minute, no matter where you are. Focusing on your breathing also gives you the opportunity to immediately change your perspective on a situation. With proper breathing, you can de-stress in the supermarket, in the doctor's waiting room, or in traffic, and no one will know what you're doing. You'll find instructions for my Abdominal Breathing technique on page 48. When you use this technique, your stomach will expand as you inhale and deflate as you exhale. At the same time, you should also feel your shoulders rising and falling with each breath. This method of slow, deep breathing creates a cascade of positive physical changes throughout your body. It can slow your heart rate, lower your blood pressure, and reduce stress-associated anxiety. A sense of calm will come over you almost right away, and you'll feel your stress begin to defuse.

Moving Forward

The time you take to prepare yourself mentally can be invaluable. If you really want to be successful on this program, plus continue to exercise regularly for the rest of your life, you need to start working from the inside out. Master the mind–body connection. Stay in the moment when you're working out and eating healthfully. Don't be surprised if you find that by the end of the next 12 days, the program has resulted in dramatic changes in your figure, as well as in your entire outlook toward getting and staying in shape. Having a beautiful body for a lifetime is your ultimate reward, and it will come into your realm of possibility when you apply, and then live, what you learn here.

The 12-Day Body Shaping Miracle Workout and Diet

CHAPTER 4

How to Reshape Your Body in 12 Days

U p until now, you've probably exercised a certain way, or not exercised much at all. Or you've been told to exercise a certain way to get the body you want. So where are the flat abs, thin thighs, and shapely butt you deserve for all your efforts? If that complaint sounds familiar, I'm sorry to tell you that what you've been doing or not doing up to this point isn't what you need to shape your body. Far from it. But now it's time to stop feeling discouraged. I'm about to share with you the five biggest exercise myths that are commonly taught in gyms and fitness centers, and in books and training guides. They're myths that are believed in and practiced. When you first read what I have to say about them, you'll think it runs counter to everything you've been doing. You'll wonder if I know what I'm talking about (I do!). Some of these myths have been a part of your exercise mindset for so long, you might not believe they're false. But if you want to change your shape and get a beautiful figure, you must let go of these myths. So it's time to first understand what these myths are, unpack them, get them out of your head, and then find out what *does* work so you can do what it takes to get the body of your dreams.

Myth 1. A Great Shape Is Created Through Full-Range-of-Motion Exercises

For background, *full range of motion* is the path of movement for a joint and muscle, from how far it can be bent (*flexion*) to how far it can be stretched out (*extension*). If you are lifting weights to improve overall conditioning, enhance sports performance, and increase flexibility, then moving joints and muscles through their full range of motion is extremely important.

However, for shaping individual muscles, full range of motion is *not* the way to go. The reason is that it typically works many muscle groups at once, possibly creating too much bulk, but does not control how individual muscles shape. Put another way, full range of motion gives you far less control over your body shape. What you will practice instead, in many cases, will be short-range-of-motion exercises. This technique makes a huge difference in your ability to lengthen and slenderize a muscle. I'll explain it more fully later in this chapter.

Myth 2. Lose Your Love Handles and Flatten Your Abs Through Core Training

Here we come to one of the biggest myths that misleads people and sends them down the wrong exercise path. You can't go anywhere in the fitness world these days without hearing about "core classes," "strengthening your core," or "core performance." But what's the real deal, and why do you need core training, anyway?

For starters, *core training* ought to refer to doing abdominal exercises such as crunches or sit-ups, pure and simple. From there, however, ab training today has gotten very gimmicky. Many fitness trainers, for example, love to have you work out on an unstable surface like an exercise ball to help you build core strength. For the most part, this approach is bogus. You'll work your ankles more than anything else by training on wobbly, unstable surfaces.

Yes, you definitely want to shape, strengthen, and shrink your abs as part of your transformation, but without doing any gimmicky core exercises. On my program, you'll learn how to get firm, flat abs by selecting basic exercises and properly executing abdominal movements. In addition, the cardio program you'll follow can help blast away fat from your waistline.

Myth 3. To Reshape Your Body, You Must Use Heavy Weights

Contrary to what many people believe, going to the gym and pumping away with heavy weights is not always the best way to reshape your body. It might make you bulkier, in fact, and it probably won't do much for those saddlebag hips you may have inherited, or that belly bulge you can't seem to lose.

What you will be incorporating on this program are exercises involving a specific form of working out that is designed to reshape your muscles—and that doesn't always mean lifting hefty weights or resistances. You'll learn a whole new style of exercising, and how to incorporate it into each of your workouts. Mastering the proper form, which is easy to learn, will give you the exact results you want. So forget the idea of heavy weights—which also increase your chance of injury—and get comfortable with the idea of proper form, which is your ticket to your desired dream body.

Myth 4. More Hours Working Out Leads to a Better Body and Great Results

This, you're thinking right now, *is a myth?* How can that be, given the hours that bodybuilders, fitness models, in-shape actresses, and other well-put-together women spend in the gym to look so perfect? But it's not true! It's not the quantity of training you do, it's the quality of training. Intense exercise sessions designed to reshape muscles and resculpt your body are the way to achieve a desirable figure.

Too much training (commonly called overtraining), on the other hand, can be hard on your body. *Overtraining* is defined as doing excessive exercise without letting your body get reasonable rest. Exercise is a stress; that's why you must give your muscles adequate rest to recover. Some consequences of overtraining include the following:

- *Ongoing muscle soreness.* It is natural to wake up feeling sore and stiff after a workout. But if that soreness sticks around for more than 48 hours, then it's a warning that you may have overtrained.
- *Repetitive trauma syndrome.* Cardio work, in particular, should not be performed every single day of the week. Your joints, ligaments, tendons, and other tissues need to recuperate or you can get symptoms of repetitive trauma syndrome, a condition caused by stress on the joints sufficient to produce chronic inflammation. If you have joint problems or other orthopedic concerns, you should definitely stick to lower-impact forms of cardio such as walking.
- *Sleep problems.* Getting too much sleep or not enough, and feeling fatigued despite a good night's sleep are all also signs of overtraining.
- *Immune system problems.* If you're getting more colds, flu, or other infections than is normal for you, your body's defenses are probably impaired, and overtraining may be one reason. Your body is screaming for rest, and if necessary will put you into a forced rest mode by making you more susceptible to annoying illnesses like colds.
- *Poor physical performance.* Overtraining can impair your physical strength and endurance, making you feel less motivated to work out.
- *Psychological reactions.* Feeling burned out, bored, depressed, irritable, or angry can be signs of overtraining, too, as long as other factors have been ruled out.

The program you'll follow on the *12-Day Body Shaping Miracle* can help you avoid overtraining—but with one important caveat. You must fuel your body with good nutrition, and not cut calories or resort to crash dieting, or else your body could possibly suffer further consequences of overtraining. Restrictive crash-type dieting doesn't help your metabolism, either. When you go on one of these diets, your metabolism regards even a moderate calorie cutback as a signal that starvation is at hand, and your body starts packing away fat in case this "famine" goes on indefinitely. Even though you're eating less food, your body starts metabolizing it more slowly—burning less for energy and storing more fat as a survival mechanism. This means you may not lose weight. In fact, it's very possible to go on a crash diet and actually gain weight. Adhering to the nutritional guidelines for your body type will accelerate your metabolism, guard against the pitfalls of overtraining, and help you look and feel great. These guidelines are covered in chapter 8.

Myth 5. No Pain, No Gain

The mantra *No pain, no gain* is a huge myth! You *will* benefit from a sensible, pain-free, moderate workout program like the one I recommend in the *12-Day Body Shaping Miracle*—and you will blast away body fat. Certainly, exercise should require some effort, but it should not cause pain or discomfort. In fact, if you experience real pain, your body is telling you to stop exercising, and you had better listen to that warning message. If you continue to feel pain during an exercise, stop and do not resume until you can do so painlessly. General muscle soreness that comes after exercising is another matter altogether. It usually indicates that you're not warming up sufficiently or that you are working out too hard or too long. Sore muscles should not discourage you from exercising, or make you stop, but they should force you to slow down. One way to minimize muscle soreness is to warm up prior to your workouts and cool down and stretch afterward.

A special note about the cardio portion of this plan: The possibility of injury is much lower with the cardio program I recommend. That's because it's low-impact exercise performed with less intensity than many other types of cardio exercise. This program generally does not produce the injuries to shins, calves, lower back, ankles, and knees often caused by repetitive, jarring movements. You'll be much more likely to continue to exercise as a lifestyle if you know you won't be sidelined by painful injuries.

Scientifically documented proof exists that remarkable changes can take place in the body in only 12 days, with the proper exercise and diet program. For example:

Reduce cardiac risk factors

Researchers at St. Helena Hospital in Deer Park, California, put 500 men and women on a low-fat vegetarian diet for 12 days. Following this short experimental period, cardiac risk factors were greatly reduced. On average, the participants' total cholesterol fell by 11 percent and blood pressure dropped by 6 percent. They also lost weight. The researchers concluded that a low-fat vegetarian diet combined with exercise is an effective way to lower cholesterol and blood pressure. While my makeover diets are not strictly vegetarian, you do eat lots of plant foods, and of course you become more active. So it stands to reason that cardiac risk factors could conceivably show some improvement.

Improve your insulin response

In a study conducted at the First Medical Faculty, Charles University, Prague, a group of obese women showed a decrease in insulinemia after only 12 days following a slimming diet and a low to moderate exercise program. Insulinemia is an abnormally large concentration of the hormone insulin in the blood. Although it has many important functions in the body, insulin is a fat-forming hormone. Too much insulin in the body is implicated in obesity.

Enhance your breathing capacity

Researchers at the University of Texas put 59 patients with severe chronic obstructive pulmonary disease (COPD) on a twice-daily program of aerobic exercise of 30 to 40 minutes' duration. After just 12 days, the participants' peak oxygen consumption increased significantly. Peak oxygen consumption measures how well you can use oxygen while exercising. An increased level of aerobic fitness was demonstrated in other indicators.

Key Concepts of Success: The Miracle Principles of Body Shaping

I realize that you're on a quest to tighten up particular areas of your body, drop some body fat, and develop an enviable shape that will never go out of style. I hear you! If your body seems flabby and shapeless right now, you need an invigorated muscle challenge—which is exactly what you'll get by following this program. Without further ado, here are the key exercise principles underlying the *12-Day Body Shaping Miracle* that you'll be using the next 12 days and beyond. Please read this section carefully, and keep these principles in mind when you exercise.

Principle 1. Use Specifically Applied Resistance

In general, *resistance training* is any form of exercise that uses additional stress to force a muscle or group of muscles to contract. It helps curb muscle loss that occurs with aging and is the most effective way to develop sleek, firm muscles all over your body.

What I utilize when training my clients is a technique called *specifically applied resistance.* This means that you apply resistance supplied by exercise bands or weights (such as dumbbells and ankle weights) to very specific areas of your figure in order to tone, firm, lift, or shape these areas. You are isolating very specific—and often small—muscles in order to effect a very particular change in them, as opposed to general weight-lifting routines that often work many muscle groups all at once, which makes it harder to control how individual muscles shape. Your individualized routine uses specifically applied resistance techniques, along with short-range movements, to give you the greatest degree of control over how your body shapes. That way, you can get the exact results you desire.

You can master this principle in three ways. First, become familiar with your training tools, including exercise bands, dumbbells, and weights. These tools have tremendous muscle-shaping power and are extremely versatile. They can replace an entire gym full of machines! Second, pay attention to the exercise instructions, particularly how to position your body. Correct body positioning places precise stress on the muscle you are targeting. Finally, really focus on the muscle you're trying to reshape, and concentrate on what you want to accomplish in terms of sculpting your body. Do not get distracted.

Principle 2. Manipulate the Resistance

How much resistance you apply to a muscle or body part makes a huge difference in its ultimate shape. Here's a look at what I'm talking about in a little more detail:

- *If you want to slim or lengthen a specific area:* Decrease the resistance you're using by decreasing the tension in your resistance bands or by decreasing the poundage of the weight you're using, and increase the number of repetitions you do. Example: Instead of doing 10 to 12 repetitions of a given exercise using medium resistance, do 15 to 18 repetitions with lighter resistance. Lower-resistance/greater-repetition work tends to give you longer, leaner-looking muscles rather than larger, built-up muscles.

- *If you want to build and increase the size of an area:* Increase the resistance you're using by increasing the tension in your resistance bands or by increasing the poundage of the weight you're using, and decrease the number of repetitions you do. Example: Instead of doing 12 to 15 repetitions of a given exercise using light resistance, do 8 to 10 repetitions using medium resistance. Higher-resistance/fewer-repetition work tends to increase the overall size of a muscle to add mass to an area. Muscle size can be added where you need extra curves. However, you do have to condition your body to handle heavier weight. To do so, start light and build to the heavier resistance.

- *If you want to tighten, lift, and firm an area:* Increase the intensity by increasing the speed at which you do the movement. Bump up the number of sets and shorten the rest time between them.

- *If you want to develop symmetry:* The term *symmetry* refers to the proportion, shape, and balance of muscle on both sides of your body. Make sure to increase the number of repetitions, sets, and resistance evenly for the right and left sides of your body. Don't push to do 10 reps with one arm, for example, if you can only finish 8 with the other. Let your weaker side catch up to your stronger side before moving forward.

Principle 3. Include Short-Range-of-Motion Exercises

Most of the exercises you'll do in your individual routine involve short range of motion. In other words, you won't take an exercise movement through its entire path from flexion to extension; in most cases, you'll stop just short of full extension. This technique allows you to hit specific areas of your body to force individual muscles to contract. *As a muscle contracts, it shapes.* This technique is thus what helps create shape in a muscle.

Recently, I trained a female celebrity who was doing lunges like crazy to trim her hips and thighs. I put a stop to that immediately, since lunges actually bulk your thighs and butt. That's right! I bet if you're like most women, you think lunges are the way to get a small, tight butt. They aren't. I've never even seen a competitive bodybuilder do lunges—they're inefficient exercises. I had this celebrity do very short-range exercises for her thighs and butt, and she was able to tighten and shrink her lower body. One of these exercises was a popular move called a Leg Extension. She learned to take the exercise through a short range of motion to give her thighs a leaner, more slender contour, adding definition without adding bulk. This also helped firm a flabby area over her knees and added tone and definition to the side of her thighs. Had she continued doing lunges, her figure would have looked completely unbalanced and out of proportion.

Another area where short-range-of-motion exercise works well is the abdominals. When working their abs, many people tend to unintentionally use other muscles, such as the hip flexors (located at the front of your pelvis and attaching to your lower vertebrae and thighbone), to complete the exercises. This diverts attention from the abdominal muscles and defeats the whole purpose of ab training. To sculpt your abs, you'll isolate them fully by using a short range of movement and contracting your abs hard while moving your body in a range of motion that is no more than 4 to 6 inches. Abdominal work is a perfect example of how short-range-of-motion exercises such as the crunch or reverse crunch can help you achieve a tighter waistline.

Don't let anyone tell you otherwise: Short-range-of-motion exercises are safe for your body (as long as you perform them correctly). Most of our normal daily activities don't take our joints through their full range of motion, anyway. So this form of exercise has benefits not only in reshaping your body, but also in making you stronger and more fit for the things you do every day. What you'll learn as you go through the *12-Day Body Shaping Miracle* is that you can change the way your body looks by changing your range of motion, along with changing your diet and doing my cardio program.

Principle 4. Work a Muscle from Various Angles

Your body has more than 430 skeletal muscles that move your bones. These muscles come in a large range of sizes, types, and functions. Generally, each muscle begins on one bone—the point of origin—and ends on another—the point of insertion. When you contract, or flex, a muscle, these points of attachment are drawn together. Skeletal muscle is composed of thousands of cylindrical muscle fibers often running all the way from origin to insertion. The fibers are bound together by connective tissue through which blood vessels and nerves run.

Because a muscle's point of origin can sometimes differ in size from its point of insertion, training muscles from various angles can greatly affect their shape. Also, some muscle groups, such as your back or your thighs, are made up of a number of smaller individual muscles with fibers running in different directions.

Understanding the basics of your muscles' points of origin and insertion and their makeup can certainly enhance your workouts. Unfortunately, though, a thorough, in-depth look at muscle anatomy would take too much time here. What you need to know instead is how to analyze your own trouble spots, then work your muscles with different exercises and different angles to optimize your body-shaping efforts. You'll get that mini-education when we get to chapter 6, where you'll learn how to design and customize a workout for your own unique body-shaping needs.

For now, just keep in mind that in order to reshape your body, it's important to challenge your muscles from multiple angles. That way, you bring more muscle fibers into the act and thus develop better shape and tone.

Let me give you one quick example before we move on—your thighs. Each thigh has three sets of muscles: your hamstring muscles in the back, your quadriceps muscles in the front, and the adductor muscles on the inside. When you look critically at your thighs, perhaps you'll notice that your inner thighs lack shape and firmness. You can correct this flaw by focusing your body-sculpting effort on that area in a way that lengthens them, firming and toning them so that they appear longer, leaner, and slimmer. Using a special resistance band exercise, all you have to do is point your toes outward at a 45-degree angle while performing the move. Something as simple as changing your body position or stance allows you to hit this muscle from the appropriate angle. You'll be amazed at how quickly your inner thighs start to take on a firmer, more attractive appearance. There are many such little-known tricks I'll show you so that you can hit your muscles from different angles and push shape into your muscles where you want it.

Principle 5. Select Body-Specific Exercises

The advantage of this program compared with other exercise programs is that it's customized to your body. For example, let's say your thighs and buttocks need slimming down. So you select specific exercises for those trouble spots, along with cardio to burn fat and slenderize your lower body. But with the *12-Day Body Shaping Miracle,* you also include building-up exercises for your shoulders to offset your larger lower body, thus giving your body more shapely contours. You add a bit here, take some away there, and before long a more balanced shape emerges. That way, out-of-shape muscle groups get extra attention. Soft spots firm up. Inches are added and subtracted. No body parts are overdeveloped or underdeveloped at the expense of others. Simply target the muscles of those areas in your workout and challenge them with the exercises you've selected. This approach can transform your figure in ways you never thought possible—better proportions, less body fat, greater muscle tone and development, and more.

Principle 6. Practice Abdominal Breathing

One of the most overlooked and relatively unknown aspects of many exercise programs is breathing. Important for success, proper breathing:

- Supplies the oxygen your muscles need to perform at maximum levels and to burn fat. If you make it a practice to oxygenate your body, you'll become trimmer and more fit, plus feel more energetic and invigorated than you have in years.

- Helps establish the mind–body connection (see chapter 3) that makes breathing a conscious act; it also helps you maintain your focus on the muscle being targeted. If you concentrate on your breathing, you can't get easily distracted from your workouts.

- Helps avoid injury during the contraction portion of an exercise. If you hold your breath, particularly while contracting a muscle, you may trigger what's known as the *Valsalva effect*—a technical name for the pressure that builds up inside your body when you hold your breath. The Valsalva effect is a potentially dangerous condition because it can impede blood flow to and from your brain, causing you to black out or, worse, suffer an aneurysm or stroke.

- Is an effective way to manage stress. We usually revert to shallow, upper chest breathing when we're anxious and under stress, but we don't have to breathe that way. Using my breathing technique helps calm the body rather quickly. You may not be able to control all the negative emotions that pass through you, or the situations that evoke them, but you *can* control how you breathe.

The specific type of breathing I endorse is based on yoga breathing. In yoga, breathing is used to help calm your mind and develop better self-awareness. Used in conjunction with exercise, it helps fan the fat-burning fire in your body to speed up the rate of your weight loss. Here's how it works:

- *Step 1.* Take a deep breath through your nose, filling your lower abdomen. Your abdomen should rise as you inhale, not your chest. Note: If your belly doesn't rise, you're breathing from your upper chest and getting less oxygen as a result.

- *Step 2.* Exhale through your mouth, pushing the air out by contracting your stomach muscles. As you do this, your abdomen should fall. Air eases in and air eases out, with a slow current of respiration that is steady. This is the natural, proper way to breathe that we forget as we grow older. Watch a baby or an animal breathe sometime, and you'll see that this is exactly how it's done. Most adult breathing is shallow and not deep enough. This method of breathing is very important to true relaxation and to establishing the mind–body connection that is so important to the achievement of your goals. Breathe deeply like this, and progressively relax your body, beginning with your feet and working your way up to the top of your head.

As you introduce Abdominal Breathing into your exercise and cardio routines, you'll be delighted to see your body shed pounds and inches steadily. At first, you'll have to concentrate on mastering this technique, but over time and with continued practice it will become a good-for-you, second-nature habit.

Principle 7. Rest Your Body to Change Your Shape

You will *not* be working out every day on this 12-day program. When you are exercising to change and shape your body, rest is essential. Your body restores itself during periods of rest. If you let yourself get overtired, or if you push your body too hard in your resistance or cardio training, you can tear muscle tissue and put your body into a state of stress. Obviously, this can be counterproductive to your goal of making over your body.

Immediately after you exercise a muscle, biochemical activities within that muscle are activated, initiating processes that lead to muscle firmness, shape, and overall development. The muscle fibers themselves have become damaged, in a way. But with adequate rest and proper nutrition, your body repairs the damage caused by the workout, then compensates by firming and developing the muscle tissue a bit more than before. The result is a positive change in your muscles—enough to create a visual difference. If you interrupt this process before it's finished, however, you may stall your progress. The general rule that you will follow is to allow a minimum of 72 hours of rest before training the same muscle or muscle group again. One exception is your abdominal muscles, which can be trained four times a week if your body requires concentrated toning work on your midsection.

Keep this in mind: Your body will change faster if you rest it! This program is generous on recuperative time so that you can maximize your progress. Once you start seeing how great you look, you'll agree that less truly is more.

CHAPTER 5

Prepping for the Next 12 Days

efore our 12 days actually begin, there are some final preparations I'd like you to make. Consider this your get-in-gear chapter, the chapter that will get your mind and body in sync, the chapter that will set the stage for your success. In this chapter, you're going to pull together everything you need in order to start changing the shape of your body. Important: Make sure you have completed the Blueprinting Questionnaire in chapter 2 so that you know your body type.

Become an Artist with Your Own Body

This is crucial: Now that you know your body type, you must go a step further. You must look at your body very critically and honestly. Then take some "before" pictures. Now, don't panic. No one has to see these but you, and they are an important tool to keep you focused on your end result. Please take these pictures. In 12 days, your body shape *will* change, and you're going to want to see this and quantify the difference. Then if you choose to continue using my methods—and I hope you do—you'll stay supermotivated to continue on your path.

I'd like you to take three pictures of yourself: one from the front, one from the side, and one from the back. (You may need a tripod to do this; or you could enlist the help of a trusted friend.) You need to see as much of your body as possible, so wear a bathing suit, preferably a two-piece. It's fine to use a digital camera or a Polaroid if you're uncomfortable about anyone seeing the photos; however, 3-by-4 prints from your photo processor are better. It's helpful to use a color copier or your computer to enlarge these photos, then print them out on plain paper so you can draw on them.

Next, get a dark pen or indelible marker to highlight the areas on your photographs that you would like to reshape. As you go through the process, take an honest, realistic look at your body.

Start at the top of your body, circling areas you want to change and making notations on what you'd like to do. For example:

- Look at your shoulders.

   Do your shoulders droop? Get rid of the droop.

   How about your posture? Is it hunched? Straighten it up.

- Look at your arms.

   Are they toned, or is there loose flesh on the back? If there is, carve it off.

- Now look at your chest.

   Is it bony or hollow? Fill it in.

   Does too much fat hang over your bra? Carve it out.

   How do your breasts look? Are they as firm and as lifted as you'd like? If not, mark this.

- What about your midsection?

   Is there too much flab around your tummy? Outline the area you'd like to reduce.

   Do you have love handles? Remove them.

- Finally, what about your lower body?

   Your buns—are they sagging? Pick them up.

   Are they too wide? Carve them down.

- How about your thighs and hamstrings?

  Are they loose and oversized or thin and undertoned? Use your pen to delineate the changes you want.

- How about your calves?

  Do they need more shape? Give it to them.

Another trick to help you visualize your best body is to find a picture in a magazine of a model or celebrity who has what you consider a great body. Use it to help you decide what areas to draw on in your pictures, and then use it as a reference every day. This will help you with your visualization exercises.

These pictures represent your best body, and you *can* achieve it. This program gives you the tools and now you have a crystal-clear picture of what you're aiming for. The closer you get to your goal, the more these pictures will help you.

Measure Up

As a benchmark, use a simple tape measure and take body-circumference measurements of key areas, specifically your abdomen, your thighs, and your hips. That way, you can watch the inches melt away as you use the exercise and diet techniques in this book.

To begin, take the following measurements using a cloth tape measure:

- Your waist measurement at your belly button.
- Your shoulder line, from the end of your left shoulder to the end of your right shoulder.
- Your chest, across your bust, from the left side to the right.
- Both thighs at their widest points.
- Your hips at their widest point.
- Both calves at their widest points.
- Both arms at their widest points.

Stand with your feet apart and your abdomen relaxed. Do not take these measurements over your clothes. The tape measure should be snug on your skin, but not constrictive.

Record these numbers in a notebook, and watch them change for the better as you begin to change your shape.

Assess your shape in this fashion at least twice—as you begin the program and after the 12 days.

Also: Please weigh yourself prior to starting the program, after you finish the 12 days, and every 6 days (not daily!) as you continue working toward your body-shaping goals. To weigh yourself, pick the same time (since weight fluctuates throughout the day due to many factors, such as food consumption and water retention), and use the same scale each time, because scale calibrations differ and each will read a little differently. All of these assessments are important and provide the benchmark against which you'll measure your progress toward a firmer, shapelier you.

Check Your Vitals

If you're starting a resistance-training program for the first time, have your blood pressure checked to rule out high blood pressure; if you do have this condition, it's important to get it under control. Please be aware that resistance training can increase your blood pressure. Should you have uncontrolled high blood pressure, you could compromise your health. Don't leave anything to chance; see your health care practitioner for a blood pressure check.

In general, a normal blood pressure reading is below 120 systolic and 80 diastolic, or below 120/80. While you may not feel any symptoms, uncontrolled high blood pressure can put you at risk for serious medical conditions. As your blood pressure numbers go above the normal range, so does your risk for having a heart attack or stroke. Every 20-point increase in your systolic (top) number or 10-point increase in your diastolic (bottom) number doubles your risk of heart attack or stroke.

While high blood pressure cannot be cured, it can be controlled. Talk to your doctor about lifestyle changes such as diet and exercise, as well as medicines, that can help lower your blood pressure. Sticking to the regimen you develop with your health care provider is the best way to keep your numbers under control.

Taking blood pressure medication may also put you at risk for low blood pressure. Most medical experts believe that a blood pressure of less than either 90 systolic or 60 diastolic (only one reading need be low) is considered lower than normal. Low blood pressure can be a cause of concern because it may signal an underlying problem, particularly when the blood pressure drops suddenly. In addition, low blood pressure can be a dangerous condition that deprives the brain and other vital organs of nutrients and oxygen. If you are taking blood pressure medication, be sure to consult your physician, especially while doing this program. Your physician should monitor your blood pressure carefully and possibly adjust medication accordingly.

While you're at it, be sure you have no pre-existing medical problems such as low blood sugar or diabetes, or use of medications like ACE inhibitors (these can cause dizziness or light-headedness during a workout), which could be aggravated by exercise. Always check with your physician before beginning any exercise program. For more information on medical conditions that may affect exercise and weight loss, refer to appendix A.

Gather Your Workout Equipment

The routines in this book employ some very basic and inexpensive exercise equipment. Dumbbells—also known as free weights—are superior for firming up muscle and building strength in the shortest possible time. A dumbbell is a short bar with iron or sand-filled vinyl plates on each end. Exercises with dumbbells work groups of muscles and do an excellent job of isolating and defining specific muscles. It's a good idea to have several sizes, or poundages, of dumbbells on hand. Remember, you don't need big heavy weights to firm, tone, or even build your muscles. Having a set of 2-pound, 3-pound, 5-pound, 8-pound, and 10-pound dumbbells is what I recommend. Most women must start with very light weights, because they don't have the same strength as men and can be injured. In fact, if you are weak or aged, a 1-pound dumbbell may be just fine for you with certain exercises.

In addition to dumbbells, please purchase exercise bands—among the most effective body-shaping tools ever designed. These employ elastic resistance so that you can apply controlled, muscle-shaping resistance precisely where you need it. Exercise bands are tubes of flexible, stretchable rubber with handles on the ends for comfort and easy use. You can use the bands to work almost any muscle group, including your triceps, biceps, chest, back, shoulders, thighs, hamstrings, abdominals, and many others. Exercise bands typically have a handle at each end and come in several different levels of difficulty, which is determined by their elasticity and color-coding. You may wish to have two or three bands on hand in order to increase your resistance. Exercise bands are great for toning and shaping, and are a convenient training tool if you must travel frequently.

Get some ankle weights, too, in poundages such as 1 pound, 2 pounds, 3 pounds, 4 pounds, or 5 pounds. These are flexible weights that can be strapped and contoured to your ankle to add a little extra challenge to your workout. Ankle weights are effective for exercises to really sculpt your leg muscles. These weights add lots of variety to your workout, and muscles respond much more quickly to a variety of exercises. Be sure to start with lighter poundages when using ankle weights. Again, if you have never trained or are weak, start very lightly with 1-pound weights.

Exercise mats are a must. For abdominal exercises and stretches, they cushion you from the hard floor. Include a stable, sturdy chair as part of your setup, too.

With these tools, you've virtually set up your very own home gym. Working out in the comfort of your own home is convenient. You don't have to spend time shuttling to and from the gym. A home workout better conforms to your schedule. What's more, the privacy factor appeals to many women. If you don't like the way you look in gym clothes, no one has to see you exercising at home. You can focus on reshaping your body without feeling inhibited.

Set up your home gym in a room with plenty of space. A room that's too crowded can be uncomfortable to exercise in and present too many possible tripping hazards.

Your exercise room should be well ventilated, too. If your air conditioner doesn't move enough air, keep it circulating with an electric fan. The optimum temperature range for working out is between 60 and 80 degrees Fahrenheit.

If possible, put up some mirrors in the room to help you check your exercise technique. Even though you might think the mirror is your worst enemy, when it comes to changing your body it can be your best friend: You can see where the muscle is contracting, and ultimately, being shaped. This instant feedback is encouraging.

Perhaps most important, your workout area should be a room you like being in. So many people make the mistake of choosing a dark corner of the garage or a dungeon-like basement. Psychologically, you won't feel like going in there. Maximize everything you can for motivation.

With a very simple home gym, you can work out anywhere, anytime, and reap enormous benefits. For example, dumbbells, exercise bands, and ankle weights will help:

- Resculpt your body.
- Develop lean muscle, which is metabolically active. (This means your muscles can burn body fat more efficiently than can untoned muscle, even at rest.)
- Iron out those dimply pockets of fat known as cellulite, thus improving overall skin tone.
- Subtract inches from your figure.

As your body begins to shift from fat to firm on the *12-Day Body Shaping Miracle*, you will start to see a curvier figure in very little time. You'll begin to look better, be more energetic, and feel more confident in your clothes.

START MOISTURIZING YOUR SKIN DAILY

When your body changes quickly, as it will on this program, your skin may not keep up. It may lose a bit of its elasticity just as you're starting to make progress in changing your shape. Who needs that, just as you're starting to eat right and work out to look and feel your best? Fortunately, you can prevent this by moisturizing your entire body every single day.

The most effective time to do this is just as you get out of the shower or bath, since your skin absorbs moisturizer best when it's warm and damp. Make this a daily ritual, although you don't have to limit moisturizing to just once a day. Do it anytime your skin feels dry. You cannot overmoisturize your skin.

What kind of moisturizer? I recommend any cocoa-butter-based formulation. A major emollient used in skin lotions and cosmetics, cocoa butter is an *occlusive,* meaning that it hydrates by forming a protective barrier over the skin to prevent moisture loss. What makes cocoa butter so moisturizing is its emollient oils, which come from the cocoa beans. Cocoa butter is also loaded with skin-protective antioxidants and countless nutrients such as calcium, potassium, and iron.

Don't worry if you can't afford the best product on the shelf. Cocoa butter is inexpensive, so you don't have to buy the most expensive or the fanciest bottle of moisturizer. Before you consider spending a fortune, rest assured that most cocoa-butter-based products will do the trick. Be sure to read the labels, however. The closer cocoa butter is to the top of the ingredients list, the more cocoa butter the product probably contains.

I am 57 years old, and I heavily moisturize my skin daily with a cocoa butter formulation. My skin looks very youthful, very tight, and very taut for my age. I don't have stretch marks, even though my skin has been subjected to the ups and downs of muscle gain due to my earlier career as a bodybuilder. Cocoa butter helps prevent stretch marks and is the reason my skin has so much elasticity. It is also effective against wrinkles. The ongoing process of moisturizing your skin will keep your skin looking young, elastic, and smooth.

One more tip: If you have very dry skin, try adding some flaxseed oil—or whatever your doctor recommends—to your diet.

Get Your Reward Ready

There is one last thing you should do. For making it through the first 12 days of this program, you want to offer yourself a (non-food-related) reward. Something really nice. Something you really want. So please: Plan now to go out and buy something to celebrate the changing of your shape by the end of the 12 days. That final day isn't far off, either. Maybe your reward is a new outfit, a shopping spree, some pampering at a day spa, a makeover, a new hairstyle. Whatever it is, you will deserve it.

Overview of the 12 Days

Consider this section a preview of coming attractions. I want you to know what's coming up so that you'll see just how easy and doable this program is. This section is your calendar, road map, and game plan all rolled into one. It tells you exactly what you'll be doing and how you'll be prioritizing over the next 12 days. Knowing what to expect will help equip and empower you for success. Just continue to believe in yourself and in this program, and each day you'll move closer to giving your body a better shape.

Day 1. The first day, you'll start off following the customized eating plan for your body type. You'll get in sync with how to eat multiple meals throughout the day, and learn how to accelerate your metabolism through this mode of eating. Today is the first day of your shape-changing workout, too, in which you'll work your lower body and midbody; start the routine you custom-designed for yourself (see chapter 6). Shoot for 45 minutes to one hour of cardio today, as well, depending on the recommendations for your level of conditioning. Your mind creates your reality. Keep the image of your dream body in the forefront of your mind.

Day 2. Continue following the food plan for your body type, so that it begins to feel like a natural way of eating. You'll do your second workout today, exercising your upper body, as well, along with cardio. You must remember that you are working on a piece of art; put your attention where it needs to go and make sure that what you're doing for these particular areas is effective. Stay focused. Review your photographs. Each day, you are taking a significant step toward your dream body.

Day 3. No resistance training today! Your third day is a day of rest. Getting enough rest is key to proper body shaping, since it is during rest periods that your muscles change and reshape. If you forgo rest days, you'll overstress your muscles, slow your progress, or, even worse, cause an injury. Don't be surprised if you start feeling lighter and more energetic already. Your body's metabolism is in the process of changing. Some people can even drop a few pounds within the first couple of days. Don't forget to drink the recommended amount of water throughout the day. Doing so will help your metabolism stay charged up. Practice positive affirmations so that you stay focused and motivated. Examples: *I have the power to change the shape of my body. I can feel my body changing. Everything I need to develop my dream body is within me. I have a healthy, beautiful body. I'm looking forward to each day of this program to experience how my figure is changing.*

Day 4. You'll resume your resistance-training routine today, working again on your lower and upper body, plus cardio. To keep meal boredom from setting in, try preparing your food in new ways. For daily reinforcement, make a list of all the positive aspects of your nutrition and workout program. Post your list on your bathroom mirror so it's the first thing you see each morning.

Day 5. Stay mentally prepared and pumped for today's workout, which targets your upper body. While changing from your work clothes into your workout wear, you're also symbolically changing into your fitness persona, like Diana Prince turning into Wonder Woman. You're not a normal woman; you're the woman who possesses beauty, strength, and many skills. Make both your workouts and your nutrition positive experiences, and they will continue to reward you the rest of your life.

Day 6. Wake up and take a few quiet minutes to reflect on achieving your dream body. Today is your second rest day—a good time to focus on healthy nutrition. Make a quick trip to the grocery store for some fresh vegetables and lean protein for this evening's dinner. Take time to notice and appreciate the colors of the fresh produce on display. Before going to bed, visualize how productive your workout will be tomorrow. You'll succeed because you've made the commitment. Never lose sight of the fact that exercise is the process of changing your body for the better.

Day 7. Congratulate yourself. You're one week into the program! Weigh yourself this morning, and expect to see a drop in your weight. Many people who do this program can lose 5, even 10, pounds the first week. Resume your workout today—again, exercising your lower body and midbody. Focus on increasing your level of effort and placing more demands on your muscles so that you can continue to change the shape of your body. Continue to trust the program.

Day 8. Today begins another week. You should see and feel the effects of eating and exercising correctly for your body type, while getting your figure closer to your desired shape. Have another great workout (upper body this time), and don't neglect your cardio. Continue to faithfully follow your meal plan. The pounds and inches should automatically be melting away. Rejoice in the fact that your clothes feel looser.

Day 9. Today is another rest day. Think about how close you are to mastering the essentials of changing your shape. You can see your figure changing, and feel your metabolism working better than perhaps it has in a long time.

Day 10. You've made a commitment to change. Congratulate yourself for that, and be proud of yourself. Keep believing in yourself and in this program. The more positive thoughts you have about yourself, the more you'll make positive decisions each and every day. Commit to another day of clean, perfect eating. Add a slice or two of cucumber to your water, or maybe some lemon slices. Enjoy your water as a special elixir you're giving your body to function at its very best. As you do your resistance-training routine (lower body and midbody), notice how much better your body looks, how much better it moves, how much better it feels. You deserve these special joys.

Day 11. Today is the next to the last day of the 12-day program. As you do your upper body resistance training and cardio, visualize even more fat melting from your body. Metabolic changes have occurred, and will continue to occur over the next 24 hours. Continue to work on your eating program; think of it as a positive tool for deflecting body fat. Begin to think how you will "keep on keeping on" beyond the initial 12 days. Outline for yourself a plan, with new goals. Maybe this involves using my kit, the *6-Week Body Makeover* (available from www.provida.com), or perhaps you've mapped out what you will eat and how you will exercise in the weeks to come in order to meet your goals. Whatever you do, start thinking about the immediate future and maintaining the momentum you've already built.

Day 12. You've been waiting for this day, I'm sure! Time for some final reflection. Is it worth 12 days of your life to start changing your shape while getting healthier? Is it? Lots of people are skeptical that significant changes can be made in 12 days. You've proved them wrong. Ask yourself how you feel at this point. I'd be very surprised if you don't want to continue eating and exercising like this after the 12 days! Be sure to weigh yourself and retake your measurements. Then stand in front of a full-length mirror and admire. Now go out and give yourself that reward for the new body you now have!

Twelve days are just a start of what should be a lifetime of being able to shape and reshape your body. As you learn and master the techniques in this book, you will begin to understand exactly how your body responds to my exercise methods as well as to proper diet. You will learn how some simple exercise principles can change the shape of individual muscles to create the exact look you desire. This program is all about developing the skills to become an artist with your own body. And that means you'll be able to make your body look any way you want and keep it that way for the rest of your life.

CHAPTER 6

Figure Fixes: Customizing Your Workout

here we are! Now comes the time when you get to custom-make a workout for yourself. Using the tools and techniques we have discussed so far, you will now shape and define each area of your body to sculpt it the way you want it to look. You will use specifically applied resistance and other techniques to isolate specific muscles and shape your body. To put it simply, you now have the tools to be an artist with your own body, to mold and sculpt it as you desire.

There are more than 25 individual exercises in this chapter, and you do not need to do all of them. Not everyone's body is alike, and not everyone wants the same results. Unlike other exercise programs you may have tried before, this one is designed specifically for you. Having completed the Blueprinting process and marked your photographs, you know exactly what areas you need to firm, tone, or shape. Pay special attention to the Blueprint Pointers in the exercise instructions; these pointers will tell you which body types and which trouble areas each exercise is designed to target.

To get started customizing your workout, use the steps that follow.

Step 1. Review Your Body Type and Trouble Spots

Look over the "before" photographs that you took and marked up. In the space below, write down your body type and list the areas of your body that you want to change and reshape, based on your photographs.

63

My body type is: _____

Areas I want to change: _____

_____

_____

Step 2. Orient Yourself to the Body-Shaping Exercises

Read through the exercises and the exercise instructions in this chapter, paying close attention to the Blueprint Pointers and the Shaping Goal listed under each exercise. This information gives you specific guidelines on how the exercise works to tone, tighten, shape, and sculpt trouble spots. Also, please pay attention to exercises that specifically address your body type. Understanding the purpose of each exercise will help you customize a workout routine just for you.

To further help you customize your routine, refer to the General Exercise Recommendations for Body Types chart on page 65. This chart lists all the exercises in this book at a glance. It gives concise information on how each exercise fixes problem areas and which exercises are appropriate for each body type.

To use this chart, first locate the column designated for your body type. All the possible exercises for your body type are noted wherever there is a symbol. Once you have located the exercises for your body type, look at the symbol next to each exercise. The symbol tells you what the exercise accomplishes. For instance, some exercises are for slenderizing; others, creating fullness. Let's say you have heavy thighs. You would thus want to select the exercise that slims your thighs, not builds them up. The symbol ▌ refers to exercises that slenderize. These symbols provide a handy way to pick the correct exercises that will target and fix your trouble spots.

GENERAL EXERCISE FOR BODY TYPES

This chart gives you an overview of which exercises may be beneficial for your body type. The codes define for you the shaping goal of each exercise. The best indicators of which exercises to select, however, are the photographs you took of your body and the areas you marked for change. Refer to those photographs as you select your exercises.

Code:

● = The exercise mainly shapes, tones, and defines.

❙ = The exercise mainly lengthens and slenderizes the muscle.

◊ = The exercise adds a bit of size and fullness to an area.

↑ = The exercise mainly lifts and shapes.

⊤ = This exercise is excellent if you need to improve your posture.

Body Types	A	B	C	D	E
Exercises					
1. Calf Raise (do not include this exercise if you have large calves)	●	●	●	●	●
2. Short-Range Hamstring Curl	❙	❙	❙		
3. Full-Range Hamstring Curl				◊	◊
4. Short-Range Leg Extensions	❙	❙	❙		
5. Full-Range Leg Extensions				◊	◊
6. Freestanding Squat				◊	◊
7. Standing Glute Squeeze	↑	↑	↑	↑	↑
8. Hip Adduction	●	●	●	●	●
9. Hip Abduction	●	●	●	●	●
10. Abdominal Contraction	●	●	●	●	●
11. Abdominal Breathing	●	●	●	●	●
12. Side Contraction (if you need to create the appearance of a slimmer waistline)	●	●	●	●	●
13. Tri-Part Chest Series—Outer Edge	↑	↑	↑	↑	↑
14. Tri-Part Chest Series—Top Edge	↑	↑	↑	↑	↑
15. Tri-Part Chest Series—Inner Edge (cleavage)	↑	↑	↑	↑	↑
16. Short-Range Biceps Curl	●	●	●		

● = The exercise mainly shapes, tones, and defines.

▮ = The exercise mainly lengthens and slenderizes the muscle.

◇ = The exercise adds a bit of size and fullness to an area.

⬆ = The exercise mainly lifts and shapes.

⊤ = This exercise is excellent if you need to improve your posture.

Body Types:	A	B	C	D	E
Exercises					
17. Full-Range Biceps Curl				◇	◇
18. Triceps Pressdown—Inner Head	●	●	●	●	●
19. Triceps Pressdown—Outer Head	◇	◇	◇	◇	◇
20. External Rotator Cuff—Standing	⊤	⊤	⊤	⊤	⊤
21. External Rotator Cuff—Seated	⊤	⊤	⊤	⊤	⊤
22. Posterior Deltoid Fly	⊤	⊤	⊤	⊤	⊤
23. Short-Range Lateral Raise (only if you have overdeveloped trapezius muscles or a thick neck)					
24. Full-Range Lateral Raise				◇	◇
25. Seated Dumbbell Overhead Press				●	●
26. Rhomboid Row	● ⊤	● ⊤	● ⊤	● ⊤	● ⊤
27. Short-Range Lateral Pulldown	◇ ⊤	◇ ⊤	◇ ⊤	◇ ⊤	◇ ⊤

Step 3. Map Out Your Customized Routine

In the chart My Customized Body-Shaping Routine on page 69, list the specific exercises that address your trouble spots, as well as your body type. For example, if one of the areas you want to work on is lifting and tightening your buns, write down the exercise called the Standing Glute Squeeze next to Buttocks. Continue to do this for each area of your body.

How many exercises should you choose per individual body part? It's really a matter of conditioning. If you have been doing resistance training continuously up to the point of reading this book, there is no set number. If you are a beginner, however, you should choose one to two exercises per body part.

The more musculature is involved in the body part, the more exercises you'll select. The back and legs, for instance, have more musculature to work than the biceps. Smaller muscles such as the biceps require only one exercise.

The exercises you select constitute your customized body-shaping routine, which you will do for the next 12 days and beyond. Perform the exercises in the exact order they are listed. You will work your body in a line, starting with your lower body and working up to your upper body.

Step 4. List the Number of Sets and Repetitions You Will Perform

On the far right-hand side of the chart My Customized Body-Shaping Routine, you'll see an area where you can record the number of sets and repetitions (reps) you'll aim for. I suggest starting out with 1 set of each exercise if you're a beginner (meaning you have never done much resistance training). If you have more experience, you may perform 3 to 5 sets of each exercise. Always use a resistance that you can handle, but one that still feels challenging. As a beginner, it's perfectly fine—as well as effective—to go as high as 18 to 20 repetitions using light resistances.

If you feel you are very overweight in an area such as your legs or arms, you may have to add more sets, reps, and exercises to achieve your desired results. This approach also applies to you if you're a Body Type D or E. Doing more sets, repetitions, and exercises can help you create more muscle in just the right places to make your body more aesthetically pleasing. When trying to change the shape of your body, you must have the eye of an artist and the sensibility to undertake an exercise routine that will achieve the shape you want, but without overdoing and straining, injuring, or re-injuring an area of your body.

One way to tell whether you're doing enough reps to push shape into individual muscles is to look for what bodybuilders call the pump. The *pump* occurs when your muscles swell up beyond their normal size—you can see this in the mirror—and become very hard as a result of blood, oxygen, and nutrients being brought into the area worked. Train an individual muscle until it gets as hard as it can. To tell whether you've reached a pump, use your fingers, squeeze the muscle, and check its level of hardness. That's the point at which you know you've done enough reps at that resistance. If your muscle goes soft all of a sudden, you've done one rep too many.

Finding the level of pump or hardness is a matter of trial and error. No two bodies are the same, and no single body is the same on any two given days. It's a difficult but doable process to get to know your own body and how much exercise (reps and sets) is necessary at any given time.

We're not over yet. Now let's discuss the days on which you'll do this routine, how to adjust your resistances for best results, and how many sets and repetitions to perform. What follows are the *12-Day Body Shaping Miracle* basics to help you get in shape faster. Read on.

Workout FAQs

How many times a week should I work out?

You will perform your routine on what I call a *2-on/1-off cycle*. This means two days of training followed by one day of rest. Then repeat the cycle. On Day 1 of the cycle, you will do lower and midbody exercises; on Day 2, you'll do upper body exercises. Working your lower and midbody on one day and your upper body on the next makes your workouts manageable time-wise and gives your body adequate time to recover and go into a change mode.

What resistances should I use?

Resistance refers to the amount of weight, or stress, placed on your muscles during an exercise in order to challenge them sufficiently to activate changes in

MY CUSTOMIZED BODY-SHAPING ROUTINE

LOWER BODY

EXERCISES	SETS To tighten, lift, and firm an area: Increase the number of sets (3–5 sets) and shorten the rest period between sets to about 30 seconds.	REPETITIONS To slim or lengthen: Use lighter resistance and more repetitions (15–18). To increase size or fullness: Use heavier resistance and fewer repetitions (8–10).
CALVES:		
HAMSTRINGS:		
QUADRICEPS (THIGHS):		
BUTTOCKS:		
INNER THIGHS:		
OUTER THIGHS:		
MIDBODY		
ABDOMINALS:		
SIDE ABDOMINALS:		
UPPER BODY		
CHEST:		
BICEPS:		
TRICEPS:		
EXTERNAL ROTATOR CUFF:		
SHOULDERS:		
BACK:		

BODY-SHAPING GLOSSARY

Targeted exercise	The specific movement you perform to shape and develop a body part—for example, a calf raise, leg extension, or lateral pulldown.
Repetition, rep	The path of an exercise from the start of the movement to the midpoint and back again to the start position.
Set	A series of repetitions.
Routine	The combination of targeted exercises performed in a certain sequence.
Resistance	The amount of weight, or challenge, used in an exercise to stress the muscles significantly for shaping.

shape and in development. When you're working out with dumbbells or ankle weights, resistance means the poundage you are lifting—whether it weighs 2, 5, 8, or 10 pounds. With exercise bands, the resistance is supplied by the thickness of the band. The thicker the band, the more challenge is applied to the muscle being worked.

When you are using weights and exercise bands on the *12-Day Body Shaping Miracle,* there are light resistances and heavy resistances. For background, a *light resistance* means that you can manage about 12 to 20 repetitions using strict form and still feel challenged; with a *heavy resistance,* you can handle 8 to 12 repetitions with perfect form and feel challenged when doing so.

With either weights or bands, you'll want to start with a level of comfortable resistance. Caution: If you've never worked out before, or haven't worked out in a long time, use lighter resistances, such as 2- or 5-pound weights or less thick exercise bands. As you continue to use weights or bands, your muscle strength will improve, and the exercises will become easier and easier. When you are ready for more challenge, simply move to a heavier weight or a more resistant (thicker) band.

The right amount of resistance to use will vary from person to person and from body part to body part. At least initially, determining the proper resistance may involve trial and error, requiring you to keep a record of each workout and how many reps and sets you did, as well as a record of the resistances you used. You'll probably need to experiment a bit to find that perfect challenging resistance. A rule of thumb, however: If you can do more than 12 repetitions but still feel challenged, then that is a light resistance. If 8 or fewer reps feel very challenging, the resistance is heavy. For each exercise, choose a resistance that's challenging enough to make you feel like you are working the muscle.

When should I use a light resistance or a heavy resistance?

This question refers to another important aspect of light and heavy resistances: Adjusting your resistance helps you achieve certain body-shaping goals. As I mentioned earlier, to give the appearance of slimming or lengthening a specific area, use light resistances (with light weights or less thick exercise bands) and a higher number of repetitions (15 to 18 reps). To add fullness and increase the size of an area, use heavier resistances (with heavier weights and thicker exercise bands) and fewer repetitions (8 to 10). Whether light or heavy, the resistance must be enough to stimulate the muscles, yet not so much that you start using sloppy form. Use poundages that let you work out in a good style, but remain challenging enough to tax your muscles.

When should I increase my resistance and/or my repetitions?

The key is to challenge your muscles to work harder each time you exercise. That means progressively upping your poundages, or doing more repetitions or even more sets. Muscles adapt very quickly to stresses placed on them. For continual progress, you must always lift more weight, try a thicker band, or do more repetitions or sets (or both) with the same resistance. You may also decrease the time between sets. Increasing your effort with each workout makes your muscles firmer, stronger, and shapelier.

How fast should I perform each repetition?

In many cases, you'll want to tighten, lift, and firm an area. You can do so by increasing the speed at which you perform an exercise and by increasing the number of sets and shortening the rest time between them.

In other cases, however, repetitions should be performed slowly, in a controlled fashion. That way, you effectively isolate the muscles being worked. Fast, jerky repetitions, on the other hand, don't isolate muscles but instead place harmful stress on the joints, ligaments, and tendons. Not only is this an unproductive way to tone muscles, but it's also a dangerous training habit to adopt—it increases your risk of injury.

How should I warm up?

Warm up with a few minutes of light cardio, such as using a treadmill or walking in place. Do a single 15- to 20-rep set of each exercise, as a warm-up, taking only as much rest as you need in order to get into position for the next movement.

How important is cardio exercise on this program?

Cardio exercise helps strip away body fat to reveal your natural shape. Generally, it's preferable to perform your cardio four to six days a week, depending on your level of conditioning. See chapter 7 for information on your cardio routine.

How Customization Works—A Sample Routine

Just to give you some extra help and insight into customizing a routine, here is how one of my clients designed her own routine, based on the steps and instructions I discussed above. Jennie's body type is B. Her overall body-shaping goal was to change her rather triangular shape into more of an hourglass. To accomplish that, she needed to slenderize her thighs, lift her buns, and flatten her tummy. Her arms were rather thin, with a lot of loose flesh—a figure flaw she definitely wanted to remedy as well. Additionally, she wanted to build up her shoulders, back, and chest in order to offset her wider hips and create more balanced proportions in her figure. Jennie's calves were already very large, in her estimation, so she didn't need to do any resistance training for her calves.

As is the case with most people, she needed to be very selective about the exercises she did. In thinking through her routine, Jennie understood that to slim and lengthen her lower body, she should use lighter resistances and more repetitions—perfect for toning and trimming. On the other hand, to add some counterbalancing fullness to her upper body, she would choose heavier resistances and fewer repetitions. This approach would also create a little more lean muscle on her body, accelerating her metabolism and burning fat. Jennie did not neglect the cardio portion of her program; she did enough cardio (four to five times a week) to start shedding the fat that was concealing her shape.

Jennie felt as though just about every area of her body needed tightening and toning, so she generally began with 3 sets of each exercise and worked up to 4. Here is how she customized a body-shaping routine for herself.

JENNIE'S CUSTOMIZED BODY-SHAPING ROUTINE

LOWER BODY—DAYS 1, 4, 7, AND 10

EXERCISES	SETS To tighten, lift, and firm an area: Increase the number of sets (3–5 sets) and shorten the rest period between sets to about 30 seconds.	REPETITIONS To slim or lengthen: Use lighter resistance and more repetitions (15–18). To increase size or fullness: Use heavier resistance and fewer repetitions (8–10).
Calves: Not needed		
Hamstrings: Short-Range Hamstring Curls	3–4 sets	15–18 repetitions per set
Quadriceps (frontal thighs): Short-Range Leg Extensions	3–4 sets	15–18 repetitions per set
Buttocks: Standing Glute Squeeze	3–4 sets	15–18 repetitions per set
Inner thighs: Hip Adduction	3–4 sets	15–18 repetitions per set
Outer thighs: Hip Abduction	3–4 sets	15–18 repetitions per set

MIDBODY — DAYS 1, 4, 7, AND 10		
EXERCISES	**SETS**	**REPETITIONS**
Abdominals:		
Abdominal Contraction	*3–4 sets*	*15–18 repetitions per set*
Abdominal Breathing	*3–4 sets*	*15–18 repetitions per set*
Side abdominals:		
Not needed		
UPPER BODY — DAYS 2, 5, 8, AND 11		
Chest:		
Tri-Part Chest Series—Outer Edge	*3–4 sets*	*8–10 repetitions/ heavier resistance*
Tri-Part Chest Series—Top Edge	*3–4 sets*	*8–10 repetitions/ heavier resistance*
Tri-Part Chest Series—Inner Edge (cleavage)	*3–4 sets*	*8–10 repetitions/ heavier resistance*
Biceps:		
Full-Range Biceps Curl	*3–4 sets*	*8–10 repetitions/ heavier resistance*
Triceps:		
Triceps Pressdown—Outer Head	*3–4 sets*	*8–10 repetitions/ heavier resistance*
External rotator cuff:		
External Rotator Cuff—Seated	*2 sets*	*15–18 repetitions*
Shoulders:		
Full-Range Lateral Raise	*3–4 sets*	*8–10 repetitions/ heavier resistance*
Posterior Deltoid Fly (for better posture)	*3–4 sets*	*8–10 repetitions/ heavier resistance*
Back:		
Short-Range Lateral Pulldown	*3–4 sets*	*8–10 repetitions/ heavier resistance*

THE 7 MIRACLE PRINCIPLES OF BODY SHAPING

1. Use specifically applied resistance to reshape and sculpt your trouble spots.
2. Manipulate the resistance (lighter resistances/more repetitions to slim or lengthen an area; heavier resistance/fewer repetitions to add shape or fullness to an area).
3. Include short-range-of-motion exercises for sculpting a specific muscle.
4. Work a muscle from its various angles.
5. Select body-specific exercises.
6. Practice Abdominal Breathing.
7. Rest your body to change your shape.

THE BODY-SHAPING EXERCISES

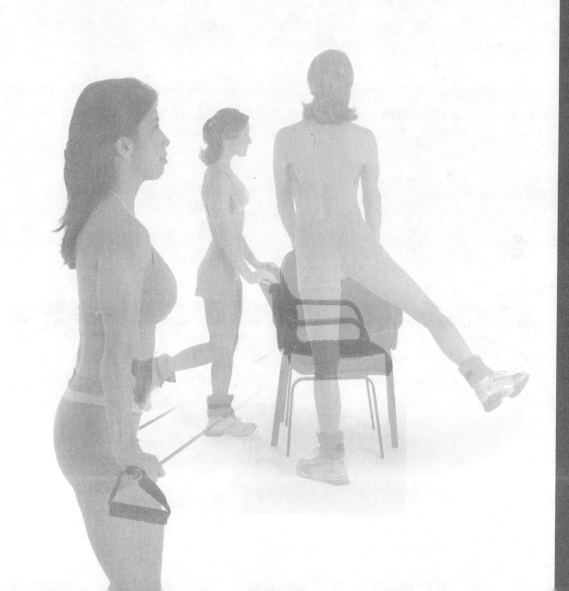

1. Calf Raise

Blueprint Pointer

This exercise is appropriate for all body types. However, if your calves are naturally muscular with some degree of shape, you do not need to include this movement in your workout routine. If you need to put tone and shape in your calves, you should start your routine with this exercise.

Shaping Goal

This exercise helps shape, tone, and define your calves without making them big and bulky. By firming this area, you develop the shape necessary to have a well-proportioned pair of legs, from top to bottom. Be prepared to show off the results of this exercise when you wear high heels!

Starting Position: Stand behind a sturdy, stable chair, placing your hands on the top of the chair's back. Keep your knees together and slightly bent forward at a 10- to 20-degree angle. The angle of your knees must not change throughout the entire movement. In other words, your knees should remain in this position. Breathe in.

Sculpting Movement: Rise up on your toes in a slow, controlled manner while exhaling. (Remember to maintain the knee position described above.) Hold the contraction for 1 to 2 seconds. Inhale as you slowly return to the start position. Repeat this exercise for the recommended number of repetitions.

MIND–BODY CONNECTION

Before you start, locate your *gastrocnemius* (calf muscle), which is the muscle shaped by this exercise. Place your hands on the backs of your knees while you are in a sitting position. Run your hands downward along the backs of your lower legs, stopping at your ankles. The muscle you have just touched is the gastrocnemius. Focus on this muscle as you do this exercise.

THE BODY-SHAPING EXERCISES

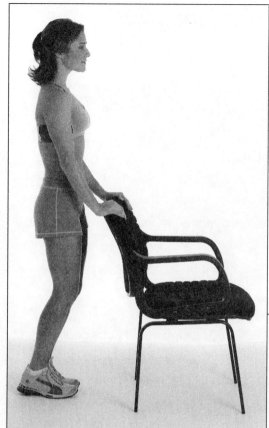

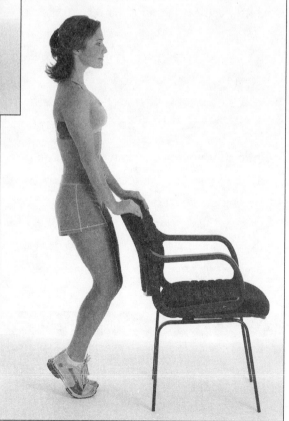

2. Short-Range Hamstring Curl

Blueprint Pointer

This exercise is effective if you are trying to lengthen, slenderize, and tone the backs of your legs. It puts a nice straight line in this area of your lower body. I generally recommend it for Body Types A, B, and C.

Shaping Goal

This is an exercise for shaping the backs of your thighs (your hamstrings). Pointing your toes straight ahead and using a short range of motion while doing this exercise will help lengthen your hamstrings while creating a leaner, more slender-looking contour and attractive definition to this area. You'll want to use a lower resistance with more repetitions to accentuate these effects. Prepare to look great in a pair of shorts as a result of this exercise!

Starting Position: Stand behind a sturdy, stable chair, placing your hands on the top of the chair's back. Begin with both feet on the floor. You will work one leg at a time. Make sure your lower back is stable. Wear a weight belt, if necessary, so that you don't injure your lower back. This is because your hamstrings attach to your glutes, which connect to your lumbar spine. On many people, the lumbar spine is one of the weakest areas. Strap 1- to 2-pound ankle weights to your ankles. Breathe in.

Sculpting Movement: Exhale as you contract your right leg upward behind you, stopping when your leg reaches a 45-degree angle. Remember to keep your toe pointed to the ground. Hold for 5 seconds. Inhale as you return your leg to the slightly raised position, as demonstrated by the model. Repeat this exercise for the recommended number of repetitions. Repeat the exercise with your left leg. If you feel pain at any time during this movement, please stop.

MIND–BODY CONNECTION

Before you start, locate the *biceps femoris* and *semitendinosus* (hamstring), which are the muscles targeted by this exercise. While you are standing, place your hands on the backs of your knees. Run your hands upward along this area, stopping at your buttocks. The muscles you are touching are your hamstrings. Concentrate on this area as you perform this movement.

The Body-Shaping Exercises

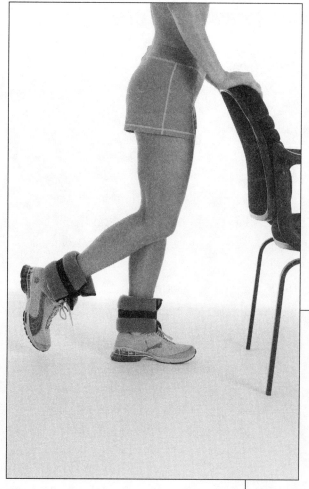

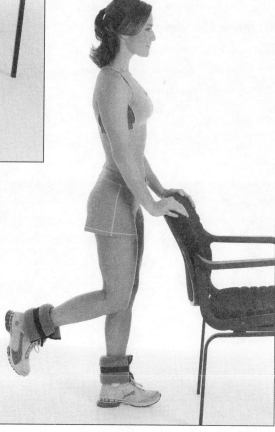

3. Full-Range Hamstring Curl

Blueprint Pointer

I recommend this version of the exercise if you need to develop more fullness in your hamstrings. Body Types C and D can often benefit from this movement.

Shaping Goal

Performing this exercise through a full range of motion adds shape and a bit of size to the backs of your thighs (your hamstrings). This gives them a slightly fuller look, with more curve and a better-defined contour. The exercise also helps firm the lower edge of your buns to help create definition between the backs of your legs and your butt. Another excellent exercise if you want to show off your legs in shorts or a swimsuit!

Starting Position: Strap 1- to 2-pound ankle weights to your ankles. Stand behind a sturdy, stable chair, placing your hands on the top of the chair's back. Breathe in.

Sculpting Movement: Exhale as you contract your right leg upward behind you, pulling your ankle all the way toward your buttocks. Hold for 1 to 2 seconds. Inhale as you return to the starting position. Repeat this exercise for the recommended number of repetitions. Repeat the exercise with your left leg. Unlike the short-range version of this exercise, your ankle should be flexed, as demonstrated by the model.

MIND–BODY CONNECTION

Before you start, locate the *biceps femoris* and *semitendinosus* (hamstring), which are the muscles targeted by this exercise. While you are standing, place your hands on the backs of your knees. Run your hands upward along this area, stopping at your buttocks. The muscles you are touching are your hamstrings. Concentrate on this area as you perform this movement.

THE BODY-SHAPING EXERCISES

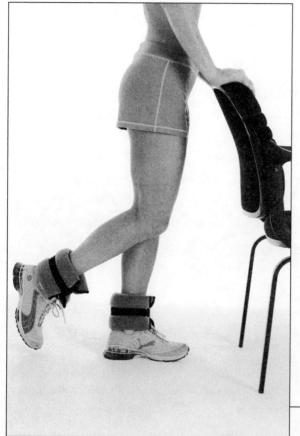

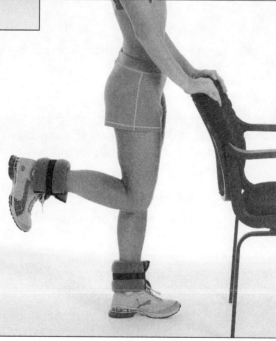

4. Short-Range Leg Extensions

Blueprint Pointer

This exercise is appropriate for Body Types A, B, and C, particularly if you need to slim and shape your thighs.

Shaping Goal

If you tend toward thick, stocky thighs, doing this exercise through a short range of motion will help lengthen the fronts of your thighs (quadriceps or quads), giving them a leaner, more slender-looking contour. Another benefit of this movement is that it helps lengthen and shape the fronts of your thighs. Use light resistance with more repetitions to accentuate these body-shaping benefits.

Starting Position: Strap 1- to 2-pound ankle weights to each ankle. Sit in a sturdy chair with your back straight and feet flat on the floor. Keep your knees and heels together. Point your toes forward. Exhale as you lift and extend your legs straight outward so that they are parallel to the floor.

Sculpting Movement: Inhale as you bring your legs downward halfway to the floor, 6 to 8 inches (depending on your level of resistance or training experience) from the starting position. Hold the contraction for up to 30 seconds. Exhale as you return to the starting position. Repeat this exercise for the recommended number of repetitions.

MIND–BODY CONNECTION

Before you start, locate the *rectus femoris*, *vastus lateralis*, and *vastus medialis*, all of which make up the quadriceps of your front thighs. Place your hands on the tops of your knees while you are in a sitting position. Run your hands along the tops of your legs to your pelvis. The muscles you have just touched are the ones being sculpted in this exercise. Focus on this area as you perform this movement.

THE BODY-SHAPING EXERCISES

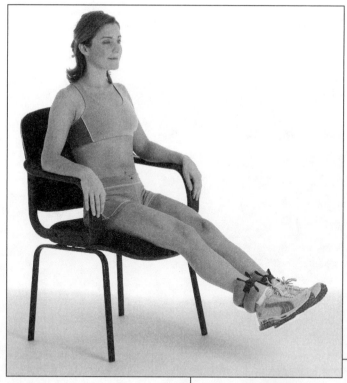

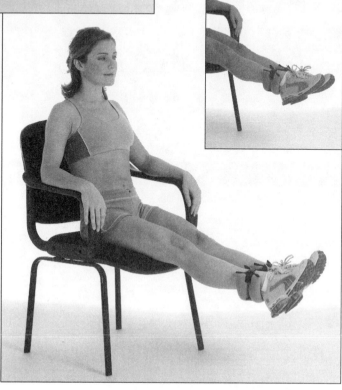

5. Full-Range Leg Extensions

Blueprint Pointer

This exercise is best for Body Types D and E, which are often characterized by lanky, formless thighs.

Shaping Goal

If you tend toward thin, shapeless thighs, doing this exercise through a full range of motion will help add shape and a bit of size to the fronts of your thighs (quadriceps or quads), giving them a slightly fuller contour. This is an effective movement if you want shapelier and firmer thighs. Another plus: This exercise helps fill in areas of loose skin on the fronts of your legs.

Starting Position: Strap a 1- to 2-pound ankle weight to each ankle. Sit in a sturdy chair with your back straight and feet flat on the floor. Keep your knees and heels slightly apart. Keep your toes back. Breathe in.

Sculpting Movement: Exhale as you raise and extend your legs straight out. Move only your lower legs to isolate the muscles of the front thigh. Keep this movement slow and controlled, without kicking your legs up. At the top of the movement, squeeze your muscles slightly as you hold the contraction for 1 to 2 seconds. Flex your ankles with your toes pointed up, as demonstrated by the model. Repeat this exercise for the recommended number of repetitions.

MIND–BODY CONNECTION

Before you start, locate the *rectus femoris*, *vastus lateralis*, and *vastus medialis*, all of which make up the quadriceps of your front thighs. Place your hands on the tops of your knees while you are in a sitting position. Run your hands along the tops of your legs to your pelvis. The muscles you have just touched are the ones being sculpted in this exercise. Focus on this area as you perform this movement.

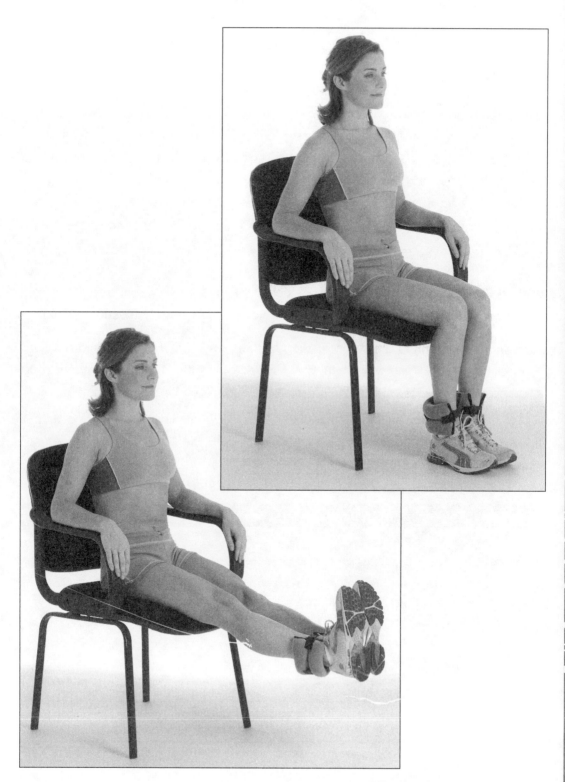

6. Freestanding Squat

Blueprint Pointer

If your thighs and hips are already larger or bulkier than you desire, do not include this exercise in your routine. This exercise is effective, however, for Body Types D and E, which usually need a bit of size and shape in their lower bodies. For general toning of this area, this is a good move.

Shaping Goal

This exercise targets your thighs, inner thighs, and hips. It's designed to shape and add a bit of fullness to these areas.

Starting Position: Stand behind a sturdy, stable chair, placing your hands on the top of the chair's back. Turn your toes slightly outward; this will help shape your inner thighs.

Sculpting Movement: In a slow, controlled fashion, lower your buttocks into a sitting position until your knees are bent at a 90-degree angle. Push back up from your heels, not your toes, to the starting position. Squeeze your buttocks together. Don't ever let your knees track over your toes; lean back slightly. Repeat this exercise for the recommended number of repetitions. If you feel any pain in your back, knees, hips, or ankles, stop immediately.

MIND–BODY CONNECTION

Before you start, locate your *gluteus maximus* (buttocks) and find the *biceps femoris* and the *semitendinosus* (the hamstring), which are the major muscles targeted by this exercise. Place one hand on your backside until you reach the area where your leg begins. Focus on working these areas as you perform this movement.

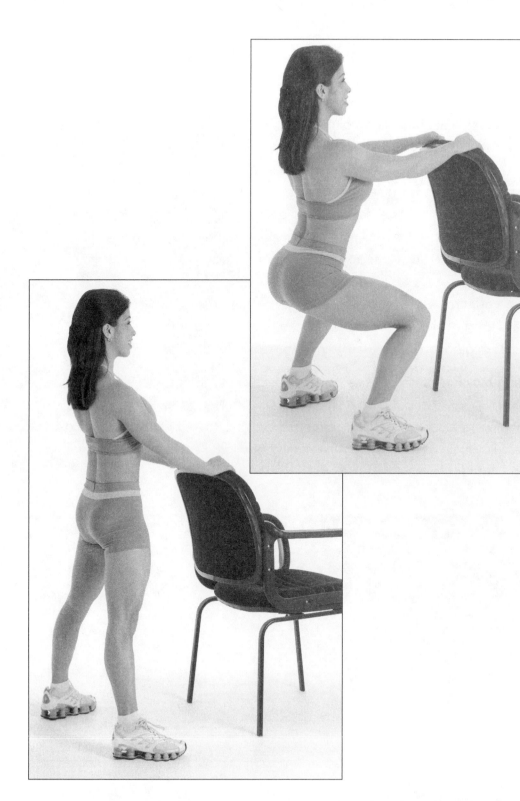

7. **Standing Glute Squeeze**

Blueprint Pointer

This movement is appropriate for all body types, particularly if you want to firm and tighten your hips and lift sagging buns.

Shaping Goal

If your buns tend to sag and need tightening, this is one of the best exercises for correcting these problems. This exercise adds shape to your glutes to give the illusion of slim hips. With this one body-shaping movement, you'll be ready to show off your strong, sexy buns in tight jeans, a swimsuit, or Daisy Duke short-shorts in no time at all!

Starting Position: With your knees slightly bent, stand behind a sturdy, stable chair, placing your hands on the top of the chair's back. Space your feet about 12 inches apart and turn your toes slightly outward. Breathe in.

Sculpting Movement: Exhale, rise up, and straighten your legs, while keeping your weight on your heels. Squeeze your buttocks together as tightly as you can, using a slight pelvic tilt. Hold this contraction for 5 to 10 seconds to lift and firm the butt. Inhale as you return to the starting position. Repeat this exercise for the recommended number of repetitions.

MIND–BODY CONNECTION

Before you start, locate your *gluteus maximus* (buttocks), which is the major muscle targeted by this exercise. Place one hand on your backside, then squeeze your buttocks together. The portion you flex is the inner portion of your gluteus maximus. Focus on working this area as you perform this movement.

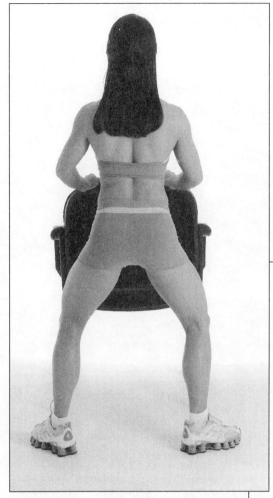

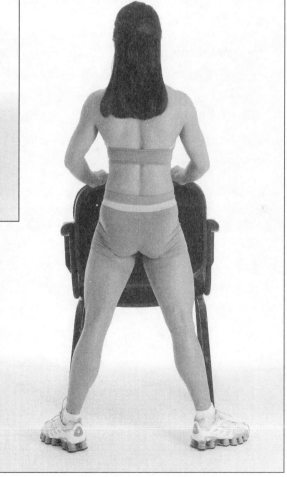

8. Hip Adduction

Blueprint Pointer

This exercise is appropriate for all body types. If you have critically assessed your figure and feel as though your inner thighs lack firmness, by all means include this exercise in your body-shaping routine.

Shaping Goal

This exercise adds firmness and tone to your inner thighs.

Starting Position: Strap a 1- to 2-pound ankle weight to each ankle. Stand behind a sturdy, stable chair, placing your hands on the top of the chair's back. Position your feet in a split stance, as pictured, with both back and front feet slightly turned out. Breathe in.

Sculpting Movement: Exhale as you extend your left leg inward at a 45-degree angle. Hold for a full second. Do not lock your knees; keep them relaxed. A short range of movement is all you need. Inhale as you return to the starting position. Re peat the exercise for the recommended number of repetitions; then repeat the movement with your right leg. If you feel any pain in your low back, inner thigh, or anywhere else during this movement, please stop.

MIND–BODY CONNECTION

Before you start, locate your *adductor* (inner thigh), which is the major muscle targeted by this exercise. Place your right hand on the inside of your left leg near your knee. Run your hand up along your thigh toward your pelvis. The muscle group you have just touched is the adductor. Focus on working this muscle group during the movement.

THE BODY-SHAPING EXERCISES

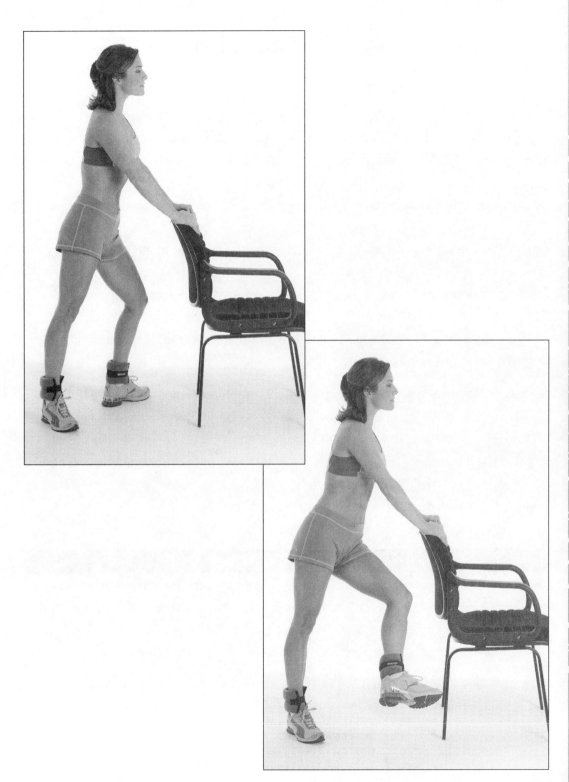

9. Hip Abduction

Blueprint Pointer

This exercise is appropriate for all body types. If you have critically assessed your figure and feel you lack tone or have saddlebags, by all means include this exercise in your body-shaping routine.

Shaping Goal

By performing this exercise with your toes pointed in, you target your body-shaping efforts on your outer thighs. The result is more shapely, better-contoured hips and thighs. This exercise is also a good way to reduce the appearance of saddlebags.

Starting Position: Strap a 1- to 2-pound ankle weight to each ankle. Stand behind a sturdy, stable chair, placing your hands on the top of the chair's back. Position your feet in a split stance, as pictured, with both back and front feet slightly turned out. Breathe in.

Sculpting Movement: Exhale as you bring your right leg straight out to the right side, creating a 45-degree angle. Hold for a full second. Do not lock your knees; keep them relaxed. A short range of movement is all you need. Inhale as you return to the starting position. Repeat the exercise for the recommended number of repetitions; then repeat the movement with your left leg. If you feel any pain in your low back during this movement, please stop.

MIND–BODY CONNECTION

Before you start, find your *gluteus medius* (the top of your buttocks) and *tensor fasciae latae* (abductor), which are the major muscles targeted by this exercise. Place your right hand on your right hip and back just over your buttocks as you stand in the starting position. Slide your hand forward to the top of your thigh. The muscles you have just touched are your gluteus medius and your abductor. Focus on working these areas as you perform this exercise.

THE BODY-SHAPING EXERCISES

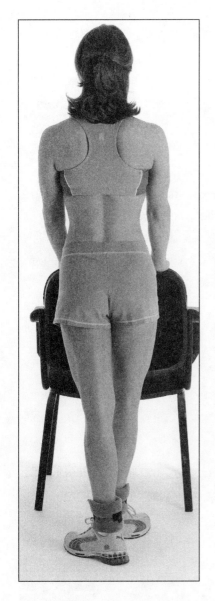

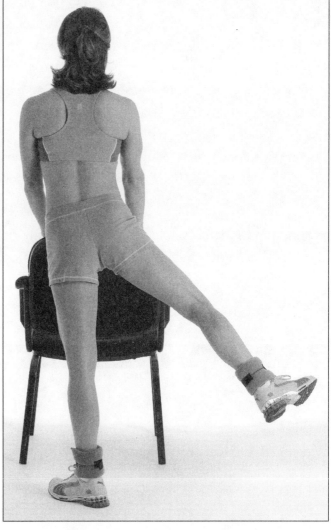

10. Abdominal Contraction

Blueprint Pointer

This exercise works effectively to create firm, flat, and sexy abs and is appropriate for any body type.

Shaping Goal

If you're dreaming about wearing low-rise jeans and a cropped shirt, this exercise is one of your best bets. Of course, you'll have to burn away most of the fat lying atop your midsection by performing long slow distance cardio (see chapter 7). But as you start to lose your belly bulge, you'll want to give your abs shape and definition. This exercise is designed to do just that—firm and flatten your entire abdominal wall—but without the pain and strain associated with sit-ups. Please note: Never work your abdominals before working your lower body. Your abs hold the integrity of your entire trunk system. If your abs are weakened when you work your legs, you could hurt your low back. If you have any type of back problem, do not perform this movement.

Starting Position: Stand with your feet about 12 inches apart and extend both arms over your head, as if you are reaching to the ceiling. Breathe in. (You can also do this exercise in a seated position.)

Sculpting Movement: Exhale as you contract your abs down and inward, creating a 10- to 15-degree angle, since the abs require only a very short range of motion (anything beyond a short range is useless). Hold this contraction for 3 to 5 seconds. Inhale as you return to the starting position.

MIND–BODY CONNECTION

Before you start, find your *rectus abdominus* (commonly called the abdominals or abs), which is the major muscle targeted by this exercise. Place your hand just above your navel in the center of your torso. Move your hand upward. Focus on the areas you have just touched as you perform this exercise.

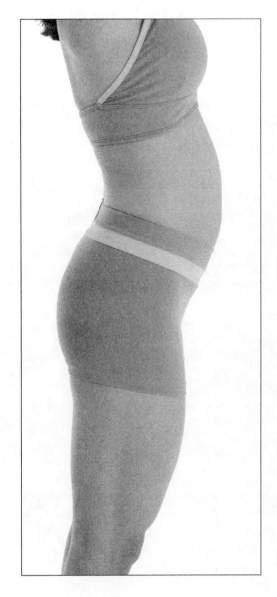

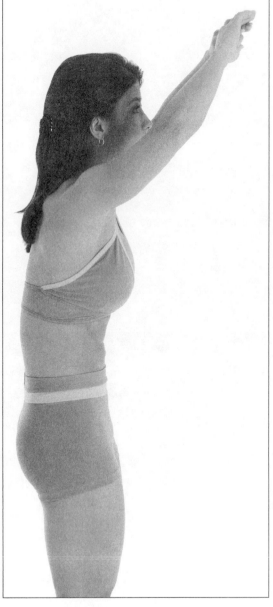

11. Abdominal Breathing

Blueprint Pointer

This is an excellent movement for any body type—one that you can do anytime, anywhere, to tone and strengthen your abdominal muscles.

Shaping Goal

This exercise is designed to firm and tighten your abs for a strong, sexy midsection. It also helps your muscles develop into a flat shape. Abdominal Breathing is a technique you should use when performing all your body-shaping exercises. It helps develop the mind–body connection.

Starting Position: Stand with your feet about 12 inches apart and extend both arms over your head, as if you are reaching to the ceiling. Inhale deeply, letting your stomach muscles naturally push out as your lungs fill with air. Do not hold in your stomach while inhaling. (You can also do this exercise in a seated position.)

Sculpting Movement: Exhale, squeezing your stomach flat to the back of your spine as you flex your stomach muscles. Inhale as you return to the starting position. Keep in mind that this is a breathe-in/stomach-out and breathe-out/stomach-in movement. It is critical to use this technique when doing other abdominal exercises.

MIND–BODY CONNECTION

Before you start, find your *rectus abdominus* (commonly called the abdominals or abs), which is the major muscle targeted by this movement. Place your hands on your stomach, 4 inches below your navel. Focus on working this area as you perform this exercise.

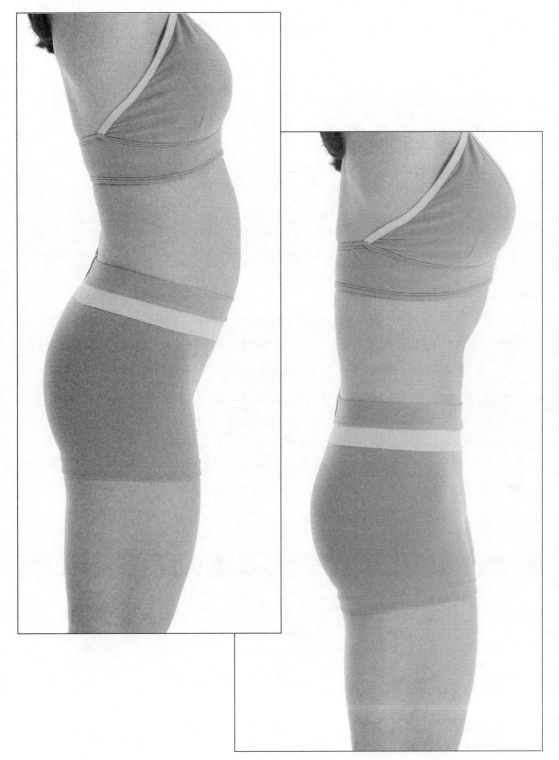

12. Side Contraction

Blueprint Pointer

While this movement is appropriate for all body types, you will want to choose this exercise if you need to pull in your love handle area or give your waist a more narrow look.

Shaping Goal

This targeted shaping move is ideal for firming and toning the muscles on each side of your body (that area between the side of your torso and your abdominals). As these muscles become firm, they tend to pull in your waist to give you a more narrow, defined waistline. Having a smaller, tighter waistline helps improve your symmetry.

Starting Position: Stand slightly pigeon-toed (toes turned inward), with your feet about 12 inches apart. Keep your chin somewhat elevated. Place your right hand behind your head with your elbow bent, as pictured. Breathe in. (You can also do this exercise in a seated position.)

Sculpting Movement: Exhale and crunch down on your right side. Your elbow should aim toward your outer heel. Tighten your stomach and squeeze your abdominal muscles. Hold this contraction for 1 to 2 seconds. Inhale as you return to the starting position. Repeat on the opposite side. Practicing Abdominal Breathing while you do this exercise will help ensure that you develop the flattest abs possible.

MIND–BODY CONNECTION

Before you start, find your *abdominal oblique* (left and right side of your lower torso), which is the major muscle group targeted by this exercise. Place your left hand on your right side, on the same level as your navel. Focus on working this area as you do this exercise.

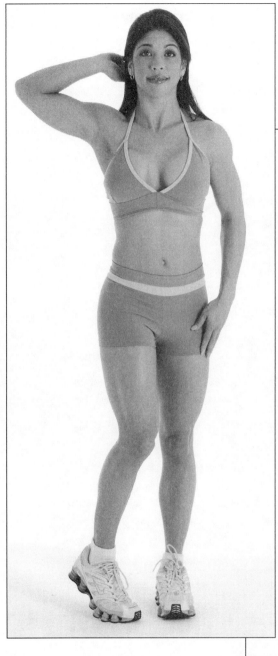

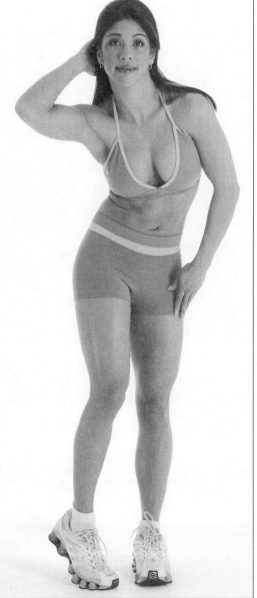

13. Tri-Part Chest Series—Outer Edge

Note: Many women would like to change some aspect of their breasts. These three exercises will help you do that, but you must do all three. This works your chest from three angles: outer, top, and inner (cleavage). Concentrating on these angles fills and lifts your chest. While these exercises won't give you a bigger bust, they will help tone and tighten the muscles underneath to give you a natural lift and, as a consequence, the look of perkier breasts.

Blueprint Pointer

This exercise is appropriate for all body types.

Shaping Goal

The first exercise concentrates on the outer chest. Firming the outer edge of your chest helps lift your bosom, adding support at the outer edge so your breasts don't sag. This movement also firms the area that tends to bulge out over your bra strap.

Starting Position: Sit in a sturdy, stable chair, with your feet on the floor. Grasp the handles of a resistance band in each hand. Have a partner stand behind you to stretch the band out beyond your shoulders. Or you can anchor the midpoint of the band around a sturdy object behind you. Start with your arms spread wide at shoulder height and slightly forward of your shoulders. Keep your elbows slightly bent. Breathe in.

Sculpting Movement: Exhale as you bring your wrists halfway in. Use a short range of motion—no more than 12 to 18 inches—in order to target your outer chest. Keep your elbows slightly bent. Hold the contraction for 1 to 2 seconds. Throughout the movement, keep your neck relaxed, chin up, and back straight to avoid pressure on your shoulders.

MIND–BODY CONNECTION

Before you start, find your *pectoralis major* (chest muscle), which is the major muscle targeted by this exercise. Place your right hand on the left side of your chest as if you were saying the Pledge of Allegiance. You should feel the outer edge of the pectoralis major near your underarm. Focus on working this area as you perform the exercise.

THE BODY-SHAPING EXERCISES

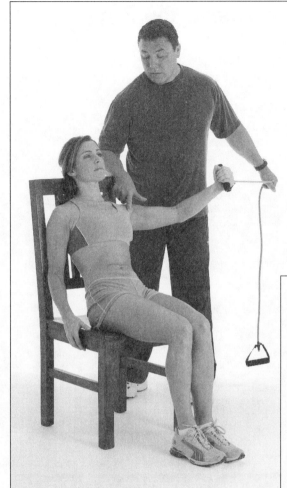

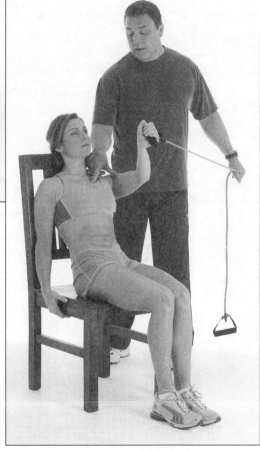

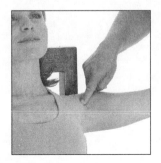

14. Tri-Part Chest Series—Top Edge

Blueprint Pointer

This exercise is appropriate for all body types.

Shaping Goal

This exercise targets the top of your chest in order to lift and support your breasts, counteracting sagging.

Starting Position: Sit in a sturdy, stable chair, with your feet on the floor. Grasp the handles of a resistance band in each hand. Have a partner stand behind you to stretch the band out behind you, as pictured. Make sure your partner has a firm grip on the band, holding it with both hands interlocked. Or you can anchor the midpoint of the band around a sturdy object behind you. Start with your arms spread in a U-shape slightly forward of your shoulders. Keep your elbows slightly bent. Breathe in.

Sculpting Movement: Exhale as you bring your wrists together, straight over your head, straightening your elbows slightly as you complete the movement. Your thumbs should be facing upward. Hold the contraction for 1 to 2 seconds. Inhale as you return to the starting position.

MIND–BODY CONNECTION

Before you start, find your *pectoralis minor* (upper chest muscle), which is the major muscle targeted by this exercise. Place your right hand on the left side of your chest as if you were saying the Pledge of Allegiance. This is the area you'll be working. Focus on this area as you perform the exercise.

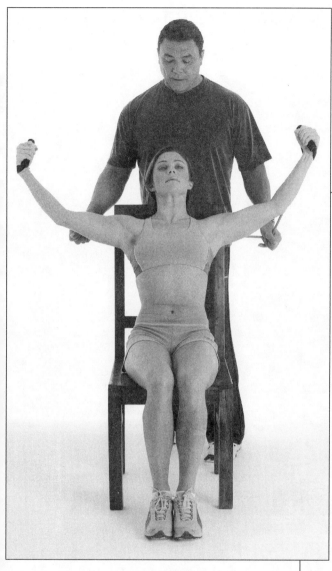

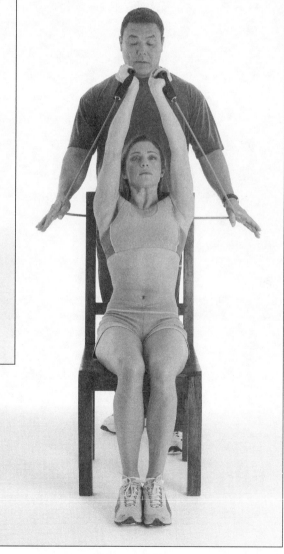

15. Tri-Part Chest Series—Inner Edge (Cleavage)

THE BODY-SHAPING EXERCISES

Blueprint Pointer

This exercise is appropriate for all body types.

Shaping Goal

This exercise firms, tightens, and defines your chest. Developing your inner chest helps increase your cleavage.

Starting Position: Sit in a sturdy, stable chair, with your feet on the floor. Grasp the handle of a resistance band in your left hand. Have a partner stand at your left side to stretch out the band for added resistance, as pictured. Or you can anchor the midpoint of the band around a sturdy object. Start with your left arm spread wide, and slightly forward of your shoulder. Keep your elbow slightly bent. Also, keep your neck relaxed, your chin up, and your back straight to avoid any strain on your shoulders. Breathe in.

Sculpting Movement: Exhale as you bring your left arm around to the front of your chest, straightening your elbow slightly as you complete the motion. Squeeze hard at this point and hold the contraction for 1 to 2 seconds. Inhale as you return to the starting position. Repeat the exercise on the opposite side.

MIND–BODY CONNECTION

Before you start, find your *pectoralis major* and *minor* (chest muscles), which are the two major muscles targeted by this exercise. Place your right hand on the left side of your body as if you were saying the Pledge of Allegiance. Move your hand to the inner edges of your chest muscles (the cleavage). The pectoralis minor is just underneath the pectoralis major. Focus on working these inner areas as you perform this exercise.

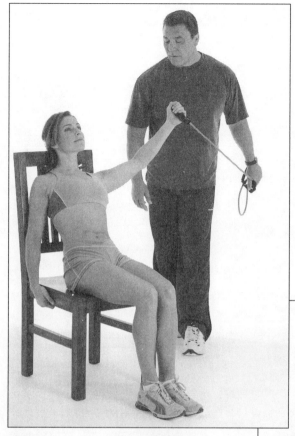

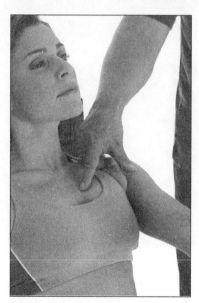

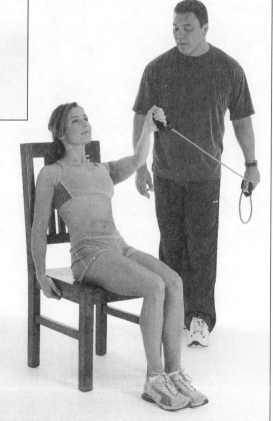

16. Short-Range Biceps Curl

This exercise is appropriate for most body types. If you are a Body Type D or E, and your arms are already long and lean, you do not want to do this exercise.

Shaping Goal

By keeping the range of motion on this exercise short, you tone the front portion of the top of your arm (between your elbow and your shoulder) without adding bulk. Instead, you sculpt long, firm, slender-looking arms that are well proportioned. The well-defined arms you'll develop will look great with sleeveless fashions.

Starting Position: Take a dumbbell in each hand, and stand with your feet firmly together on the floor. Keep your arms down at your sides, with your wrists pointed forward. Lock your elbows in front of your hips. Bend your knees slightly to take pressure off your lower back. Keep your neck relaxed and your chin up to keep tension off your back. Breathe in.

Sculpting Movement: Exhale as you flex your arms at your elbows and pull your wrists straight up toward your shoulders. Stop just before your forearms are parallel with the floor. Contract your biceps partially—just a few inches up. Hold the contraction for 1 to 2 seconds. Inhale as you return to the starting position.

MIND–BODY CONNECTION

Before you start, find your *biceps* (the front of your upper arm), which is the major muscle targeted by this exercise. Put your right arm in the starting position. Place your left hand just above your right elbow on the front of your arm. As you flex your arm, you will feel tension in your biceps between your elbow and shoulder. Focus on working this area when you perform this exercise.

THE BODY-SHAPING EXERCISES

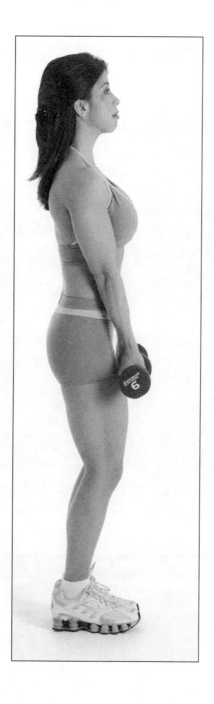
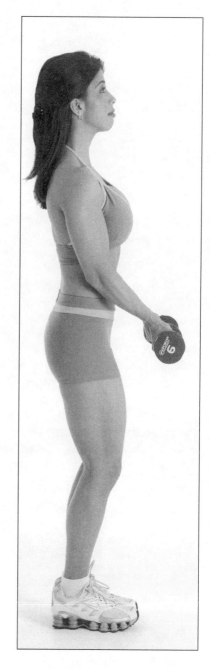

Figure Fixes: Customizing Your Workout   107

17. Full-Range Biceps Curl

Blueprint Pointer

This exercise is most appropriate for Body Types D and E, who tend to have lean arms, or for Body Types A and B if the arm area is flabby. What's more, this exercise is terrific for building strength to carry groceries, luggage, even your kids.

Shaping Goal

Using a long range of motion on this exercise helps fill out the front portion of the top of your arm between your elbow and your shoulder. This exercise will give your arms a firmer and more developed shape, along with a bit of size. Besides, well-defined arms always look terrific with sleeveless fashions.

Starting Position: Take a dumbbell in each hand, and stand with your feet firmly together on the floor. Keep your arms down at your sides, with your wrists pointed forward. Lock your elbows in front of your hips. Bend your knees slightly to take pressure off your lower back. Keep your neck relaxed and your chin up to keep tension off your back. Breathe in.

Sculpting Movement: Exhale as you flex your arms at your elbows and pull with an upward arc toward your shoulders. The palms of your hands should face the ceiling. Pause for a moment to contract your biceps at the peak of the exercise. Hold the contraction for 1 to 2 seconds. Inhale as you return to the starting position.

MIND–BODY CONNECTION

Before you start, find your *biceps* (the front of your upper arm), which is the major muscle targeted by this exercise. Put your right arm in the starting position. Place your left hand just above your right elbow on the front of your arm. As you flex your arm, you will feel your biceps contract, bunching up between your elbow and shoulder. Focus on working this area when you perform this exercise.

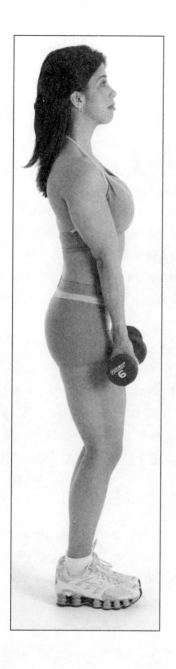

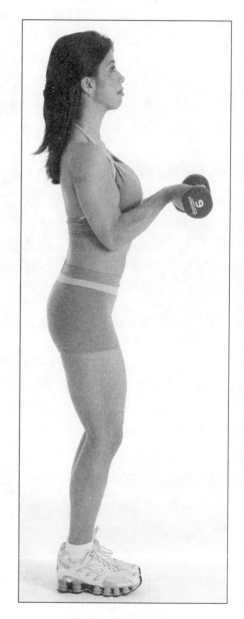

18. Triceps Pressdown—Inner Head

Blueprint Pointer

This exercise is effective for anyone who wants to tone and tighten the backs of the upper arms. Body Types D and E can use this exercise to develop more fullness and shape in their triceps, while Body Types A, B, or C can use it if the area is loose and flabby.

Shaping Goal

This exercise firms and tones that often loose and flabby area at the back of the arms (the triceps). It specifically targets the inner head of the triceps to create fullness. Performing this exercise correctly can tighten up the backs of your arms, adding firmness and tone without making them too bulky. With arms that are toned and defined, you can go sleeveless with confidence.

Starting Position: Stand with your feet about 12 to 18 inches apart and grasp the handles of the resistance band with an underhanded grip, palms up. Have a partner anchor the band, or secure it to a stable object at an angle. Keep your upper arms locked at your sides, with your arms bent at about a 90-degree angle. Keep your knees slightly bent—to take pressure off your lower back—and your shoulders down. Also, lift your chin slightly to avoid creating tension in your back or neck. If you feel any pain in your back, neck, or wrist, stop the exercise immediately. Breathe in.

Sculpting Movement: Exhale while pulling the handles downward and away from you until your arms are straight down at your sides, with your wrists locked and back, as demonstrated by the model. This is very important in order to get the triceps to contract correctly. Hold this position for 1 to 2 seconds. Inhale as you return to the starting position.

MIND–BODY CONNECTION

Before you start, find your *triceps* (the back of your upper arm), which is the major muscle targeted by this exercise. Put your right arm in the starting position and place your left hand on the back of your right arm just below your armpit. As you move to the sculpting movement position, you will feel the triceps on the very back of your upper arm. Focus on working this area as you perform this exercise.

THE BODY-SHAPING EXERCISES

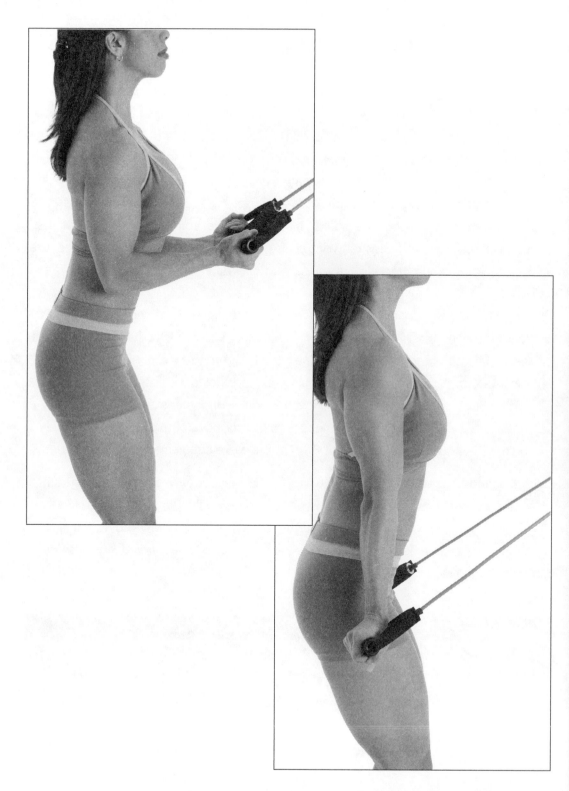

19. Triceps Pressdown—Outer Head

Blueprint Pointer

This exercise is effective for anyone who wants to tone, tighten, and define the backs of the upper arms. Body Types D and E can use this exercise to develop more fullness and shape in their triceps. Body Types A and B can use it if the area is flabby.

Shaping Goal

By doing a slight variation on the previous exercise, this motion targets the outer head of the triceps, which is the portion most noticeable from a straight-on view. It's all in the grip: Turn your hands outward and you isolate this area. This is an effective exercise if you want to create more shape and fullness in your upper arms.

Starting Position: Stand with your feet about 12 to 18 inches apart and grasp the resistance band just above the handles, with your wrists facing each other. Have a partner anchor the band, or secure it to a stable object at an angle. Start with your upper arms locked at your sides, bent so that they are parallel to the floor. Keep your knees slightly bent—to take pressure off your lower back—and your shoulders down. Also, lift your chin slightly to avoid creating tension in your back or neck. If you feel any pain in your back, neck, elbow, or wrist, stop the exercise immediately. Breathe in.

Sculpting Movement: Exhale while pulling the handles downward and away from you until your arms are straight down at your sides, with your wrists locked. As you press down, turn your wrists away from each other and downward so that your palms are facing the floor. Hold this position for 1 to 2 seconds. Inhale as you return to the starting position.

MIND–BODY CONNECTION

Before you start, find your *triceps* (the back of your upper arm), which is the major muscle targeted by this exercise. Put your right arm in the starting position and place your left hand on the back of your right arm just above your elbow. As you move to the sculpting movement position, you will feel the triceps on the side of your upper arm. Focus on working this area as you perform this exercise.

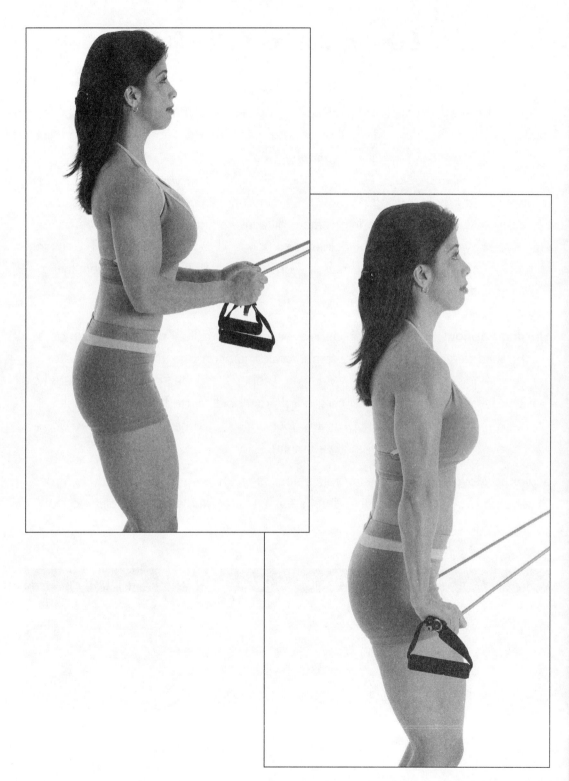

20. External Rotator Cuff—Standing

Blueprint Pointer

This exercise is effective for all body types. However, if you have or have had a rotator cuff injury, do not perform this exercise without consulting your physician first.

Shaping Goal

Although the *external rotator cuff* is a small muscle group in your upper back, it plays a large role in creating good posture. By firming and strengthening these muscles, you'll pull your shoulders back into a more attractive squared-off look—very important if you have rolled-forward shoulders or if you tend to hunch forward. The rotator cuff is one of the most neglected muscle parts. Exercising it can help prevent future problems with your shoulders.

Starting Position: Make sure you do this exercise with a light resistance, such as a 1-pound dumbbell, since the external rotator cuff consists of small muscles that don't require a lot of force to work them properly and they can tear quite easily. Stand firmly on the floor, and hold a light dumbbell (1 to 3 pounds) in each hand, with your palms facing down. Your arms should be at a 90-degree angle to your body, shoulder height. Breathe in.

Sculpting Movement: Exhale and rotate your arms up toward your head. Hold for 1 second. Do not extend farther than is comfortable. Inhale as your return to the starting position.

MIND–BODY CONNECTION

The *supraspinatus* (rotator cuff) is a group of four muscles that encircle the shoulder joint like a cuff. Before you start, find the rotator cuff, which is the major muscle group targeted by this exercise. Reach your left hand behind your back to feel beneath your right shoulder blade while in a standing position. The rotator cuff is the small muscle group in your back in this spot. Focus on working this area as you perform this exercise.

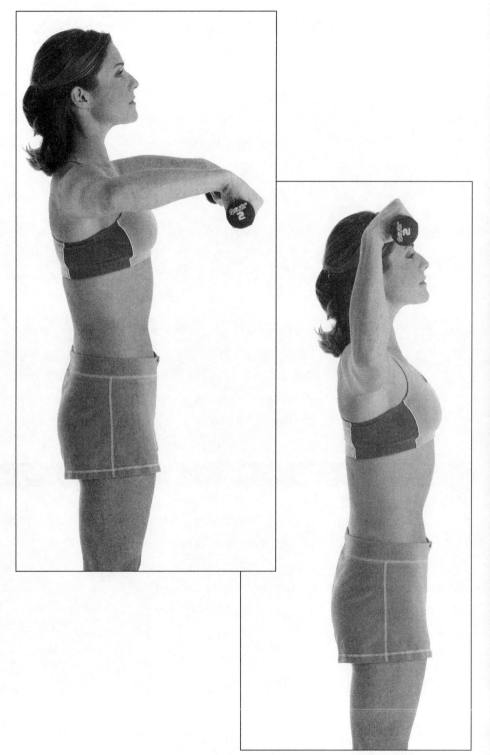

Figure Fixes: Customizing Your Workout   115

21. External Rotator Cuff—Seated

Blueprint Pointer

This exercise is effective for all body types. However, if you have or have had a rotator cuff injury, do not perform this exercise without consulting your physician first.

Shaping Goal

This is another version of the previous exercise; it helps improve your posture, plus shapes and defines your shoulders.

Starting Position: Sit in a sturdy, stable chair and grasp a light dumbbell in each hand. The rotator cuff muscles are very small, so be careful not to use too much resistance or do too many repetitions. Lean forward slightly while keeping your chest up. Tuck your elbows to your sides. Breathe in.

Sculpting Movement: Exhale and raise your arms out to your sides, until your arms are halfway between the starting position and shoulder height, as pictured. Hold this position for 1 second. Do not extend any farther than is comfortable. Inhale as you return to the starting position. Stop if you feel pain in your lower back, neck, upper back, or anywhere else.

MIND–BODY CONNECTION

The rotator cuff is a group of four muscles—*supraspinatus, infraspinatus, teres minor,* and *subscapularis*— that encircle the shoulder joint like a cuff. Before you start, find the rotator cuff, which is the major muscle group targeted by this exercise. Reach your left hand behind your back to feel beneath your right shoulder blade while in a standing position. The rotator cuff is the small muscle group in your back in this spot. Focus on working this area as you perform this exercise.

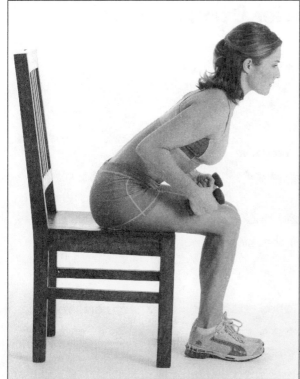

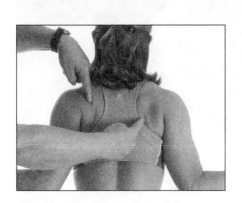

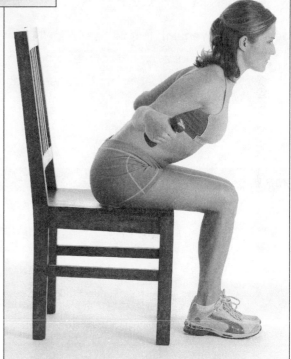

22. Posterior Deltoid Fly

Blueprint Pointer

This exercise is effective for all body types, particularly if you have a hunched-over posture, with your shoulders drooping forward, and you need to lift and straighten your shoulders.

Shaping Goal

Targeting the muscles at the back edges of your shoulders, this exercise is a great sculpting move that can dramatically improve your posture. Firming and strengthening these muscles help pull your shoulders back to give you a more upright and square-shouldered physique. Once your shoulders take on more tone, you'll look great in off-the-shoulder tops.

Starting Position: Stand with your feet about 12 to 18 inches apart, and your knees slightly bent. With your arms extended out in front of you, grasp the ends of a resistance band so that it is taut. Keep your chin up or else the tops of your shoulders (trapezius) will get worked instead of your posterior deltoid. Breathe in.

Sculpting Movement: Exhale as you pull your arms back, keeping them parallel to the floor. Squeeze your shoulder blades together. Hold this contraction for 1 to 2 seconds. Throughout the motion, keep your arms relaxed and slightly bent; do not lock your elbows. Inhale as you return to the starting position. Stop this exercise immediately if you feel any pain.

MIND–BODY CONNECTION

Before you start, find your posterior deltoid, which is the primary muscle targeted by this exercise. Hold your right arm extended in the starting position. Cup your left hand over your right shoulder with your fingers just touching the start of your underarm. Pull your right elbow back into the sculpting movement position and feel the small rope of muscle that becomes dominant as your arm bends. Focus on working this area as you perform this exercise.

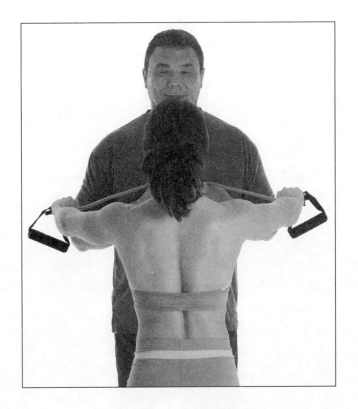

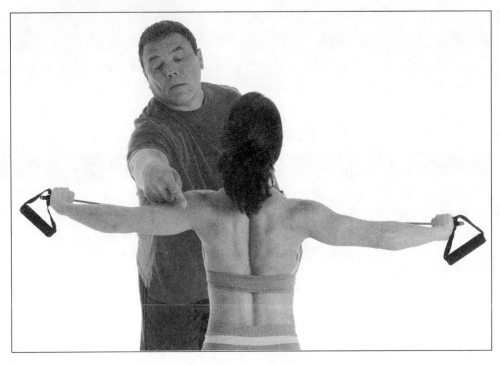

Figure Fixes: Customizing Your Workout   119

23. Short-Range Lateral Raise

Blueprint Pointer

The trapezius is either of two flat, triangular muscles of the shoulders and upper back that are involved in moving the shoulders. This move is appropriate for anyone with an overdeveloped trapezius. Often the result of stooping over a computer, this can have a dramatic effect on your posture and the appearance of your upper body.

Shaping Goal

This exercise shapes and tones the sides of your shoulders. Keeping this movement short firms, shapes, and adds definition to your shoulders and the shoulder cap without adding bulk. Additionally, this movement is especially effective if your trapezius is overdeveloped. By keeping your resistance light and doing a higher number of repetitions, you will create sleek, sexy shoulders in no time. However, do not do this exercise if you have bursitis, or a rotator cuff or neck injury.

Starting Position: Stand with your feet close together. Grasp a dumbbell in each hand and hold them with your arms resting at your sides. Keep your elbows slightly bent. Keep your neck, back, and shoulders relaxed. Breathe in.

Sculpting Movement: Exhale as your spread your arms, lifting straight out about 10 to 24 inches from each side of your waist. Hold this position for 1 to 2 seconds. Inhale as you return to the starting position. Stop this exercise immediately if you feel any pain.

MIND–BODY CONNECTION

Before you start, find your *lateral deltoid* (the top of your arm), which is the primary muscle targeted by this exercise. Place your right hand midway between your left elbow and shoulder. Begin to raise your left arm up to the side. Feel the muscle on the outside of your shoulder; this is the lateral deltoid. Focus on working this area as you perform this exercise.

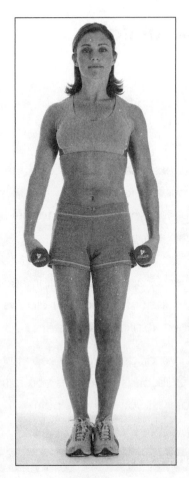

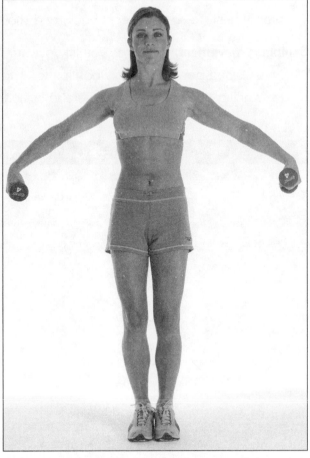

Figure Fixes: Customizing Your Workout   121

24. Full-Range Lateral Raise

Blueprint Pointer

This exercise is a good move for Body Types D and E, particularly if you have narrow, underdeveloped shoulders.

Shaping Goal

If you tend toward narrow or sloping shoulders, this exercise will help correct that trouble spot. It targets the muscles at the sides of your shoulders and at your shoulder caps to give you a bit more width and height for better symmetry and proportion. In one simple move, it can make you shapelier and more confident.

Starting Position: Stand with your feet close together. Grasp a dumbbell in each hand and hold them with your arms resting at your sides. Keep your elbows slightly bent. Keep your neck, back, and shoulders relaxed. Breathe in.

Sculpting Movement: Exhale as you lift your arms to shoulder height. Keep your wrists turned down. Hold this position for 1 to 2 seconds. Inhale as you return to the starting position. Stop this exercise immediately if you feel any pain.

MIND–BODY CONNECTION

Before you start, find your *lateral deltoid* (the top of your arm), which is the primary muscle targeted by this exercise. Place your right hand midway between your left elbow and shoulder. Begin to raise your left arm up to the side. Feel the muscle on the outside of your shoulder; this is the lateral deltoid. Focus on working this area as you perform this exercise.

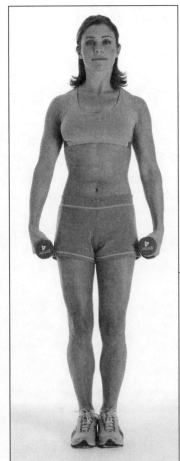

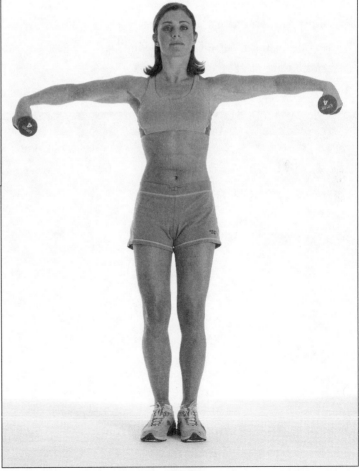

25. Seated Dumbbell Overhead Press

Blueprint Pointer

This is an excellent exercise for Body Types D and E, particularly if you'd like more size, shape, and width in your shoulders.

Shaping Goal

Whether you want to bare your shoulders in a halter top or lift luggage into the overhead compartment when you travel, this move will help develop the lateral and anterior heads of your shoulder muscles for a sculpted look.

Starting Position: Sit in a sturdy, stable chair. Grasp a dumbbell in each hand and hold the weights at shoulder level, as pictured. Breathe in.

Sculpting Movement: Exhale as you slowly press upward until your arms are nearly straight. Keep your elbows slightly bent. Inhale as you slowly lower your arms back to the starting position.

MIND–BODY CONNECTION

Before you start, cup your right hand over your left shoulder joint. The *deltoids* (shoulder muscles) are the ones targeted by this exercise. These muscles have three heads: The anterior head moves your arm up, forward, and in; the lateral head lifts your arm to the side; and the posterior (rear) head moves your arm back and rotates it out. Focus on working these muscles as you perform this exercise.

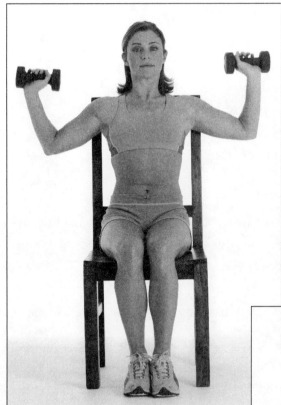

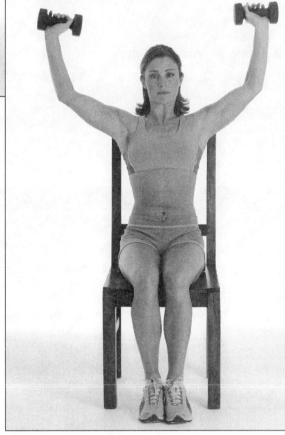

26. Rhomboid Row

Blueprint Pointer

This exercise is appropriate for all body types to create a buff, beautiful back.

Shaping Goal

This exercise targets the muscles of your midback. By activating the muscles in this area, you will help pull your shoulders back for better posture, define your middle back, and get your back in sleek, sexy condition for those backless fashions.

Starting Position: Sit on a stable stool, chair, or bench with your feet spaced apart for good balance. Have a partner hold the resistance band at its midpoint, making it taut, as pictured, or secure the band to a sturdy structure. Grasp one handle in each hand with your elbows bent and thumbs pointing up. With this exercise, it is very important to keep your neck relaxed by tilting your chin up slightly. Breathe in.

Sculpting Movement: Exhale as you pull your elbows back toward each other to your sides, keeping your arms parallel to the floor. Squeeze your shoulder blades together. Hold this contraction for 1 to 2 seconds. Inhale as you return to the starting position. If you feel pain in your mid- or lower back or neck, stop this exercise immediately.

MIND–BODY CONNECTION

Before you start, find your *rhomboids*, the muscles that pull your shoulder blades inward and the primary muscle group targeted by this exercise. Squeeze your shoulder blades together and feel the contraction of your rhomboids—the middle of your back. Focus on working this area as you perform this exercise.

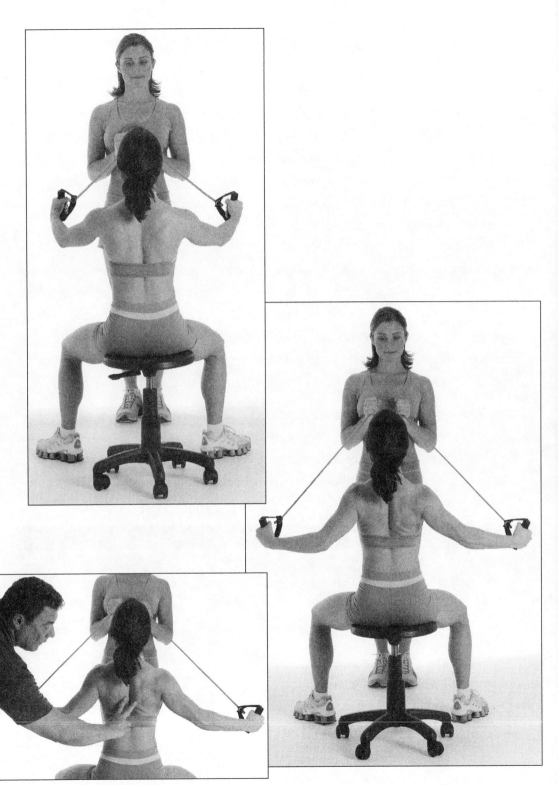

27. Short-Range Lateral Pulldown

Blueprint Pointer

This exercise is effective if you are aiming for a V-shape to help minimize the waist and hips. Body Types A and B can benefit greatly from this move.

Shaping Goal

This move is designed to target the muscles on the side of your back and under your arms. It will enable you to stand up straighter and add width to your upper body, making your waist and hips appear smaller.

Starting Position: Sit on a sturdy, stable chair, stool, or bench. Position your thighs so that they are parallel to the floor and your feet are flat on the floor, positioned directly under your knees. Have a partner stand behind you and hold a resistance band at its midpoint to tighten the band for better resistance, or anchor the band to a stable structure. Grasp the handles. Keep your arms relaxed but slightly bent at the elbows. In addition, keep your abs tight and your neck long. Breathe in.

Sculpting Movement: Exhale as you pull the band down, while letting your elbows come forward slightly in front of your body as you lift your chest. Pause and squeeze the sides of your back and underarm area. Hold that contraction for a second or two. Slowly extend your arms to begin returning the handles to the starting position.

MIND–BODY CONNECTION

The largest muscles in your back are the *latissimus dorsi* (lats), which is the primary muscle group targeted by this exercise. The lats run from just behind each armpit to the center of your lower back, and their main job is to pull your arms toward your body. As you do this exercise, focus on using these muscles to do the work rather than relying on any other muscle group.

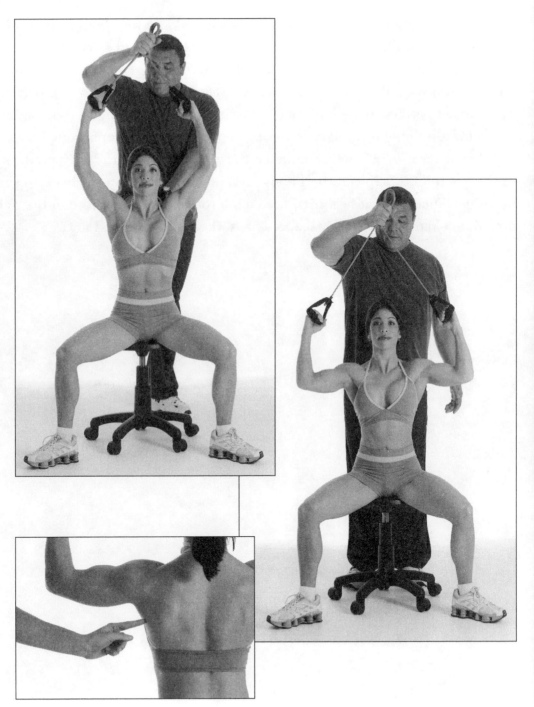

There you have it. For 12 short days, you will work out your body from head to toe, right side and left, using exercise bands, dumbbells, and ankle weights, in a routine that you custom-designed for yourself. Before long, those trouble spots—the particular regions of your body that never seem to measure up to your personal standards of perfection—will become a distant memory, as long as you continue to use these training tips and exercises to get a buffed, well-proportioned body.

There is more to it than that, however. You will also ease into a results-producing cardio routine to help you shed body fat, and you will begin to clean up your nutritional intake to eat healthier, streamline your figure, and move in the right direction toward a better body shape. That's where we're headed next.

CHAPTER 7

Cardio Meltdown

hen Hollywood celebrities or *Extreme Makeover* clients have to trim down pronto, they contact me to whip them into shape pronto. Now you can do the same—as long as you add cardio exercise into the mix to blast away the fat that is obscuring your natural figure. After all, why reshape your figure if you're going to hide it under a layer of fat?

What this portion of the program challenges you to do is several days of cardio a week, depending on your level of conditioning and experience. It is generally recognized that the best advances (especially in terms of fat loss) are made by doing cardio at this level of frequency. It will be well worth the effort: You'll rapidly begin to see the difference in how your clothes fit, and you'll start looking leaner and more toned.

So before you shudder at the thought of that much cardio, be reassured that you do not have to complete sweat-dripping sessions or endless aerobic dance classes to burn fat. Let me explain. Some of the most vigorous types of cardio—stair climbing, elliptical machines, aerobic dancing, step classes, rowing machines, kickboxing, and power-cycling (Spinning) classes—do very little to incinerate fat. Here's the reason: Intense, pavement-pounding cardio tends to burn mostly sugar, because you're recruiting muscle fibers that call on glycogen for their source of fuel. Glycogen is a form of sugar stored in your muscles, liver, and bloodstream. When your body is burning sugar, it is *not* burning fat.

The secret for shifting your body into a fat-melting mode is less intense cardio exercise performed consistently. It's a form of exercise called *long slow distance cardio,* and it includes purposely paced (not intense or strenuous) walking, slow jogging, treadmill exercise, or stationary bicycling, performed 45 to 60 minutes at a stretch. The beauty of long slow distance cardio is that it activates fat burning by utilizing muscle fibers that use fat for their fuel source, not sugar. This way of exercising aerobically is actually the most successful way to coerce your body into burning fat and is one of the workout methods I use with all my clients, as well as with the people who appear on ABC's *Extreme Makeover.* Employed during the *12-Day Body Shaping Miracle,* long slow distance cardio cranks up fat burning and helps you walk or jog off pounds and inches so that you will begin to see a dramatic body transformation by the end of this 12-day period.

Because it's not grueling or overly vigorous, long slow distance cardio should leave you feeling energized afterward, not tired. If you're feeling worn out after a cardio workout, you've pushed too hard. Sweat doesn't always mean you've busted your buns, although it can. The amount of sweat you produce usually has to do with your core body temperature, the temperature of the room you're in, and genetics, rather than your actual exertion.

Long Slow Distance Cardio May Actually Spot-Reduce Your Waistline

Long slow distance cardio just happens to be one of the best moves for creating sexy abs. It's true! With cardio (and the right diet), you can knock off abdominal fat more easily than fat elsewhere on your body. Researchers at the Washington University School of Medicine in St. Louis, Missouri, put a group of men and women, aged 60 to 70, on an exercise program that consisted of walking or jogging. On average, the subjects exercised 45 minutes several times a week. By the end of the study, both the men and the women had lost weight. But get this: Most of their weight was shed from the abdominal area. This all goes to show that a simple exercise program of long slow distance cardio can melt off abdominal fat, which creeps on us as we get older.

More spot-reducing proof: In another study, 13 obese women exercised moderately for 90 minutes four to five times a week for 14 months. At the end of the study, the women underwent CT scans to detect any changes in their deposits of body fat. Interestingly, more flab was lost from the abdominal region than from the midthigh, proving that abdominal fat is easily burned with a consistent, long-term cardio program.

Why does long slow distance cardio shrink the abs so effectively? Compared with other fat storage sites on the body, your abdominal region is lipolytically active. This means it gives up fat easily, particularly in response to cardio exercise. Cardio boosts the output of the hormone adrenaline. One of adrenaline's jobs is to increase fatty acids in the bloodstream so that your body can use them for fuel. Fat cells in the abdominal area happen to be very sensitive to adrenaline. In response to exercise, they liberate fatty acids quite readily. It's much easier to work off fat from the abs than it is from the thighs and hips, where fat cells are more stubborn. Bottom line: Cardio is a great tool to help you lose your belly bulge, if that's an area of concern on your figure.

Further, based on available evidence, the best flab-busting cardio for your midsection appear to be walking, jogging or running, stationary cycling, or treadmill exercise. Those are exactly the forms of cardio recommended on this program.

Other Cardio Benefits That Never Quit

In general, any form of cardio, including long slow distance cardio, increases special fat-burning enzymes in the body, plus builds the number and density of tiny structures in cells called *mitochondria,* where fat and other nutrients are burned. The more mitochondria you have, the more fat your body can burn.

Cardio exercise fights fat *during* exercise as well. About 20 minutes into your cardio session, your body really begins to mobilize fat. So for fat loss, you must try to work out with cardio longer than 20 minutes. Your body does not start accessing fat for fuel until 20 to 30 minutes into cardio exercise. This level of cardio also conditions your heart and lungs. The more aerobically fit you are, the sooner your body switches over to fat stores, and the greater the percentage of fat you'll burn for fuel. An aerobically fit body is a fat-burning body.

But there are many more benefits in store over the long haul: If you make a 100 percent commitment to long slow distance cardio as a part of your lifestyle, it can help normalize your blood pressure, elevate your mood, reduce tension, offset the declining metabolic rate normally associated with aging, and protect you against heart disease and possibly breast cancer.

Why Long Slow Distance Cardio Burns Fat: The Muscle Fiber Connection

In the past, you've probably exercised your buns off, but without getting very good results. All that huffing and puffing, and you're still having trouble getting into your clothes. I've heard your frustration before —which is why I designed this cardio program of long slow distance exercise so that you can blast away pounds and inches.

There's another physiological reason why this form of exercise works so effectively to target body fat, and it has to do with the composition of your muscle. On average, the human body is one-half muscle—*voluntary muscle* used for movement, *smooth* or *visceral muscle* that lines various organs, and *cardiac muscle* that helps govern the pump action of your heart. They all operate the same general way—by contracting and relaxing. This occurs because the muscle fibers, which are bundles of contracting units that make up the muscle, can shorten their length by 30 to 40 percent.

When you exercise, you use your voluntary muscles, those that move the skeleton's bones in response to the brain's conscious will. There are three types of fibers present in voluntary muscle tissue: *fast-twitch fiber, medium-* or *middle-twitch fiber,* and *slow-twitch fiber.* Depending on your body type, you may have more of one kind than another. Nonetheless, muscle fibers are highly *plastic*—in other words, they can alter their characteristics according to the type of exercise you perform. That means you can make all of these muscle fibers work for you—and mold your physique to the body of your dreams. Let's take a closer look at what I'm talking about.

Fast-Twitch Fiber—the Strength Muscle

When you swing a golf club, lift a barbell, throw a baseball, or sprint, you recruit fast-twitch muscle fibers. These fibers contract quickly, providing short bursts of energy required for explosive movements. This type of muscle fiber does not burn fat. Instead, the primary energy source for fast-twitch muscle fibers is blood sugar stored in the muscle cells themselves, as well as in the blood and liver. Although fast-twitch muscle fiber is the strength fiber, this energy source is quickly depleted, which is why a sprinter must rest after 50 to 100 yards, and a bodybuilder must rest between each set of exercises. In fact, a fast-twitch muscle fiber will give out after about 30 seconds of continuous contraction.

Fast-twitch muscle fiber is dense and hard, giving the body a muscular look. Weight lifters, football players, sprinters, and bodybuilders tend to develop an abundance of fast-twitch fibers in their musculature. When you lift weights or do other forms of resistance training, fast-twitch fiber is one of the fibers you'll use to shape, tone, define, and strengthen your body.

Medium- or Middle-Twitch Fiber—the Everyday Muscle

Medium- or middle-twitch fiber is very similar to fast-twitch fiber, in that it is also involved in explosive types of activity. However, it's also capable of longer periods of activity and doesn't have quite the strength capacity of fast-twitch fiber. When you use many of the cardio machines in the gym, take aerobics classes, or play basketball, you're using middle-twitch fibers. These are movements requiring explosive high-intensity activity but not of the quick, forceful nature of lifting a heavy weight repeatedly for 30 seconds. Like fast-twitch fiber, middle-twitch fiber burns sugar; it does not burn fat. Medium-twitch muscle fiber can be developed through resistance-training and body-sculpting exercises.

Slow-Twitch Fiber—the Fat-Burning Muscle

For fat burning, slow-twitch fiber takes on a more dominant role. Slow-twitch fiber is your body's fat-reducing fiber. This type of fiber gets most of its energy from burning fat for fuel, in conjunction with oxygen, contracting very slowly but having the ability to endure over extended periods of activity. Recruited when endurance is needed, slow-twitch fiber is very fatigue-resistant, utilized predominantly during the performance of nonexplosive cardio exercise. This fiber has only a limited ability to increase in size, and as such little, if any, muscular growth can take place.

Long-distance runners, long-distance cyclists, marathon runners, and similar endurance athletes tend to develop a greater percentage of slow-twitch fiber. That's why these athletes are generally very lean and sinewy. They utilize their body fat as fuel, burning it during a process known as the Krebs cycle. Through the Krebs cycle, your body metabolizes fat into energy. But this cycle doesn't kick in until you've done at least 15 to 20 minutes of long slow distance exercise. This creates a slow but steady demand for more energy. The body then taps into its fat stores and combusts that fat for fuel to satisfy the demand. Basically, the goal in long slow distance exercise is to use as much slow-twitch muscle fiber as possible, for as long as possible, so that you can dramatically accelerate the rate at which your body burns fat.

Making It Work: Your 12-Day Cardio Program

Now that we've looked at the science behind why long slow distance cardio works, it's time to make it work for you. To help you start reshaping your body in 12 days, I've designed this workout program to not only help you burn fat but also help you become more aerobically fit. Of course, when you use it in conjunction with your customized diet plan, you can expect to see the pounds and inches melt off. Quick results are certainly the best motivation, and the *12-Day Body Shaping Miracle* delivers them.

Ready to get going? Keep reading and let's continue. Here are the steps to making it happen.

Step 1. Choose Your Activity

For success, it's important to find activities that work for you. If you hate the treadmill but love walking outdoors or around an indoor track, these latter activities will be more effective for you. Don't walk up hills, however; only on flat ground. Of the following forms of long slow distance cardio, choose one, or two, that you enjoy and can stick with for life.

Paced Walking

Walking is a do-anywhere activity that anyone can do, and it's easy, convenient, and inexpensive. What's more, it just happens to be one of the most effective fat-burning workouts there is—as long as you do it rhythmically. I call this Paced Walking. The idea is to keep your pulse within a certain range for an extended period of time, without much fluctuation, in order to burn fat (this is explained below). Paced Walking is the perfect choice if you are out of shape, or have done little or no cardiovascular exercise in the past.

Some other important tips:

- Wear comfortable clothes, a good pair of sturdy, well-cushioned walking or running shoes, and a watch with a second hand, a stopwatch, or a heart rate monitor.
- Keep your head level as you walk and look straight ahead.
- Bend your elbows at about a 90-degree angle and keep them close to your sides. Swing your arms backward and forward as you walk.
- Let your heel strike the ground first, then roll from the heel to the ball of your foot. Push off with the ball of your foot for more momentum.
- Take comfortable, smooth strides, and try to work in your Fat-Burning Zone (see page 141).
- Warm up prior to exercising, and make sure you cool down afterward. This helps prevent injury and maximizes the oxygen uptake by your muscles for accelerated fat burning.
- Do not walk on hilly terrain. Stay on flat ground; this ensures that you use your slow-twitch muscle fibers and that your heart rate stays consistent and steady.

- To minimize the risk of injury, avoid walking on hard pavement such as concrete; stick to softer terrain like grass, footpaths, dirt, rubber tracks, and so forth.
- Make sure your walking path is safe and well lit, and let other people know your route. Carry a noisemaker or whistle. Wear reflective clothing if you exercise outside before sunrise or after dark.
- Stop and check your pulse every five to six minutes to stay in your Fat-Burning Zone. If your heart rate is too fast, slow your pace. If it's too slow, push yourself a little harder.
- Turn your walk into a meditation. Notice your surroundings or repeat a mantra, such as *I feel wonderful . . . this is the best thing I have ever done for my body.*

Walk/Jog

If you're already a walker, now might be a good time to pick up the steam with a walk/jog. This means alternating between a walk—within your target range—and a slow jog to keep your heart rate where it needs to be. What I've found to be most effective for people who are ready to push a little harder is to walk rhythmically for five minutes, followed by slow jogging for five minutes.

This sequence is a form of cardio interval training, which alternates short bursts of higher-intensity exercise with intervals of slower activity. Interval training releases hormones that create lean muscle, burn fat, and work neglected muscle fibers. All exercise helps your metabolism, but interval training gives you an extra fat burn. Your metabolic stove will burn hotter, allowing you to burn fat along the way.

For best results, continue this pattern of interval cardio for 45 to 60 minutes (preceded by a warm-up and followed by a cool-down). A walk/jog is the perfect bridge to the next level of intensity—jogging. Follow the same pointers I've given for walking and for jogging.

Slow Jogging

If you've become so good at your walking workouts, but the scale never budges, it may be time to cover some new ground with jogging. When you advance to slow jogging, expect to see results very quickly. I have found slow jogging to be the most effective method for fat burning, particularly if you want to begin trimming your hips, thighs, and buttocks.

Even so, jogging can be one of the hardest exercises on the musculoskeletal system and can increase the risk of injuries such as twisted and sprained ankles, low back problems, shin splints, knee injuries, and muscle sprains. To reduce these risks, wear proper shoes, stay on soft terrain such as grass, dirt, or rubber tracks, and make sure to warm up first and cool down afterward. Here are some additional guidelines for slow jogging:

- Maintain good posture, with your head and chin up.
- Keep your elbows bent in a 90-degree angle and held close to your side. Let your arms swing backward and forward as you jog.
- Take fairly short steps, letting your heel strike first.
- Wear sturdy, well-cushioned running shoes.
- Jog in well-lit areas and let people know your route. Wear reflective clothing if you jog at night.
- Jog on smooth, well-cushioned tracks, rather than on hard pavement.
- Monitor your heart rate to make sure you stay in your Fat-Burning Zone.
- Do not jog if you have back, knee, ankle, or foot problems, or any sort of cardiovascular disease.

Running

If you've been jogging but want to take it up a notch, because you are very conditioned, you may want to try running. Here are some other pointers for running:

- Wear sturdy, well-cushioned running shoes.
- Run in well-lit areas and let people know your route.
- Run on smooth, well-cushioned tracks, rather than on hard pavement.
- Maintain good posture, with your head and chin up.
- Keep your elbows bent in a 90-degree angle and held close to your side. Let your arms swing backward and forward as you run.
- Take fairly short steps, letting your heel strike first.
- Remember to take your pulse before your run, during it, and afterward.

Treadmill

Treadmills provide an ideal way to do your long slow distance walking or jogging indoors, at home, or in a gym. With treadmill exercise, it's easy to keep your pace constant and maintain your heart rate at the level at which your body will burn fat for energy. Also, most treadmills have some cushioning in the tread, which will reduce the impact on your joints. Motorized treadmills are preferable to manual because they keep the pace steady. Manual treadmills can force you to work too hard. Follow these guidelines for treadmill exercise:

- Start slowly to warm up. After five or six minutes, step off the treadmill to check your heart rate. To avoid injury, don't try to check your pulse while on the machine. If your heart rate is too slow, crank up the speed on the treadmill. If it's too fast, turn it down.
- Do not adjust the grade or slope of the treadmill. Instead, adjust the incline as flat as it will go. Inclined treadmills can place stress on your lower back and may also cause you to work too hard to burn fat.
- To burn more fat, try swinging your arms while you walk on the treadmill. Research shows that vigorous arm swinging increases your fat-burning potential by 50 percent, plus giving your upper body a good workout.
- Don't forget to monitor your heart rate.

Stationary Bicycle

A popular means of long slow distance exercise, the stationary bicycle is a good fat burner and overall fitness enhancer. It increases your lower body tone and enhances your aerobic power, provided you exercise consistently in your Fat-Burning Zone. Here are some tips to help you effectively burn fat:

- Adjust your seat position so that your knees have a slight bend when your legs are fully extended. Improper seat height can place undue stress on your joints.
- Round over the handlebars to take the pressure off your lower back and increase circulation in your legs.
- If the seat is too hard or narrow, invest in a pair of padded cycling shorts or get a good gel seat cover.

- Use light tension with very little resistance so that the wheels spin easily and you can keep your body in the fat-burning realm.
- Avoid programs that have you going up and down hills; stay level so that you don't miss out on the fat-burning benefits of stationary bicycling.
- Don't opt for stationary bicycling if you have very large legs, since this form of long slow distance exercise may build up your legs. Choose walking or jogging instead; these activities are more effective for slimming and toning your legs and hips.
- Stationary bicycling can be tough on the hips, lower back, ankles, and knees if you're not accustomed to this form of exercise. If it hurts, don't do it! If you can't adjust the machine to make it comfortable, go back to walking or jogging.

Step 2. Find Your Fat-Burning Zone—and Stay There!

The next important step in setting up your long slow distance cardio program is to determine your Fat-Burning Zone. This is the heart rate at which your body burns fat. If the rate at which your heart is beating is too slow during exercise, your efforts will have little fat-burning effect. If your heart rate is too fast, you'll end up burning sugar that is present in the bloodstream (glucose) and less fat. With higher-intensity exercise, your body needs to acquire fuel quickly in order to fuel your fast-twitch muscle fibers; thus, it draws from sugar stores. Your goal, then, is to get your heart rate in the zone that exists between "too slow" and "too fast" so that your body will burn proportionally more fat than sugar. When you exercise in this zone—your Fat-Burning Zone—you give your body more time to break down stored fat and use it as fuel. Using slow-twitch fiber for 30 to 60 minutes is the only exercise that burns fat; all other forms of exercise burn sugar (glycogen).

So what is your personal Fat-Burning Zone? One way to find out is to use a common formula for estimating your maximum heart rate; you then calculate a percentage of your maximum to define your Fat-Burning Zone. This zone is commonly defined as 50 to 65 percent of your maximum heart rate, or all the way to

70 percent if you are well conditioned. To calculate your Fat-Burning Zone, use the following formula:

- Subtract your age from 220 to find your maximum heart rate. Let's say you're 35 years old. Your maximum heart rate would be 185 beats per minute.
- Multiply your maximum heart rate by 50, 55, 60, 65, or 70 percent to find your Fat-Burning Zone. Using the same example, your Fat-Burning Zone would be 102 (185 x .55), 111 (185 x .60), or 120 (185 x .65).

Ideally, the closer you are to 65 or 70 percent, the better. However, if you're very heavy, out of shape, or otherwise deconditioned, you should start at 50 percent of your maximum heart rate. (As you continue exercising aerobically beyond the 12-day period, you'll want to gradually work your way up to 65 or 70 percent of your maximum.)

If you're math-challenged and hate arithmetic, use the heart rate chart below. Just find your age, and move across to the column to locate the range you're after.

HEART RATE CHART				
AGE	50%	55%	60%	65%	70%
18–19	101	111	121	131	141
20–21	100	110	120	130	139
22–23	99	109	119	129	138
24–25	98	108	118	127	137
26–27	97	107	116	126	135
28–29	96	106	115	125	134
30–31	95	105	114	124	132
32–33	94	103	113	122	131
34–35	93	102	112	121	130
36–37	92	101	110	120	128
38–39	91	100	109	118	127
40–41	90	99	108	117	125

AGE	50%	55%	60%	65%	70%
42–43	89	98	107	116	124
44–45	88	97	106	115	123
46–47	87	96	104	114	121
48–49	86	95	103	113	120
50–51	85	94	102	112	118
52–53	84	92	101	111	117
54–55	83	91	100	109	116
56–57	82	90	98	108	114
58–59	81	89	97	107	113
60–61	80	88	96	105	111
62–63	79	87	95	104	110
64–65	78	86	94	103	109
66–67	77	85	92	101	107
68–69	76	84	91	100	106
70–71	75	83	90	99	104
72–73	74	81	89	98	103
74–75	73	80	88	96	102
76–77	72	79	86	95	100

Important note: If you are already in very good cardiovascular condition, you are capable of working at 70 percent of your maximum target heart rate.

To make sure you're in your ideal fat-burning range while exercising, take your pulse by placing your middle and index fingers on the inside of your wrist. Hold them there until you feel the beating of your heart—that is, your pulse. Once you have it, simply count the beats for 10 seconds (use a watch with a second hand or a stopwatch), then multiply that number by 6 to get your heart rate for a minute. Another option for keeping tabs on your heart rate is to invest in a heart rate monitor, a handy piece of technology that costs between $100 and $300.

If your heart rate is slower than where you should be, speed up. If it's faster, slow down to get back in your Fat-Burning Zone. When you're in your zone, you should be breathing a little harder than usual, but still be able to comfortably carry on a conversation without gasping for air. If you continue to use long slow distance cardio after the *12-Day Body Shaping Miracle*, you'll develop a sense of the proper pace for your body and won't have to check your heart rate so often. Even so, you should continue to check periodically to make sure you're burning the maximum possible fat.

When it comes to melting fat, the longer you work out, the better! Realistically, you don't start burning much fat until you keep your heart rate in your Fat-Burning Zone for at least 5 to 10 minutes, and you don't start burning fat *rapidly* until after being in that zone for 30 minutes.

So the central idea of long slow distance cardio is to work out aerobically for a longer duration than normal—45 to 60 minutes—at a lower intensity, maintaining your heart rate in the prescribed zone, in order to activate your slow-twitch muscle fibers and utilize more fat for fuel. During the *12-Day Body Shaping Miracle*, you should exercise four to six times a week. That should be your goal for maximum results. Here is a suggested workout schedule:

SUGGESTED LONG SLOW DISTANCE CARDIO SCHEDULE

DAY	EXERCISE	WARM-UP + EXERCISE + COOL-DOWN
1	Paced Walking, walk/jog, slow jogging, treadmill, or stationary bicycle	45–60 minutes
2	Paced Walking, walk/jog, slow jogging, treadmill, or stationary bicycle	45–60 minutes
3	*Rest*	
4	Paced Walking, walk/jog, slow jogging, treadmill, or stationary bicycle	45–60 minutes
5	Paced Walking, walk/jog, slow jogging, treadmill, or stationary bicycle	45–60 minutes
6	*Rest* or Paced Walking, walk/jog, slow jogging, treadmill, or stationary bicycle	45–60 minutes
7	Paced Walking, walk/jog, slow jogging, treadmill, or stationary bicycle	45–60 minutes
8	Paced Walking, walk/jog, slow jogging, treadmill, or stationary bicycle	45–60 minutes
9	*Rest*	
10	Paced Walking, walk/jog, slow jogging, treadmill, or stationary bicycle	45–60 minutes
11	Paced Walking, walk/jog, slow jogging, treadmill, or stationary bicycle	45–60 minutes
12	*Rest* or Paced Walking, walk/jog, slow jogging, treadmill, or stationary bicycle	45–60 minutes

One additional point: An excellent indicator of your aerobic fitness is your heart rate at rest. In a very highly trained aerobic athlete, the heart beats 30 to 40 times a minute at rest; 70 to 80 beats a minute for normal people; and 80 to 100 beats a minute for the sedentary and out-of-shape. Check your heart rate occasionally when you get up in the morning. If it's low, your heart is beating fewer times, but pumping more blood with each beat. That means it's working more efficiently.

Step 3. Schedule Your Cardio for Optimum Fat Burning

Anytime you can fit long slow distance cardio into your schedule is the best time! For fat burning, however, some times are better than others—like after your last meal, because you can burn everything off. It has been my experience and observation that you can drop fat rapidly if you do your cardio after your last meal. In fact, researchers have found that exercising aerobically between one and three hours after a meal burns up to 15 percent more calories than if you just plop down on the sofa after eating. If your schedule permits, try that approach.

Another recommendation is to perform cardio after doing your sculpting routine. Stored glucose and glycogen supply the energy you need during your sculpting routine. But afterward, you have less of these energy sources available. When you do your cardio *after* sculpting, your primary fuel source then becomes fat—exactly what you want to burn. However, don't do this if you have hypoglycemia or are very out of shape.

Step 4. Always Warm Up and Cool Down

Before beginning your exercise program, prepare your body for the activity with a proper warm-up. Warming up increases the flow of blood to your muscles and connective tissue, causes a gradual elevation in your heart rate, increases the temperature of your active muscles for a better supply of oxygen, and positively affects the speed of muscular contraction. Basically, the warm-up readies your body for action and reduces the possibility of muscle injury and soreness later.

The best way to warm up for long slow distance cardio is simply to begin your routine, but at a slower, easier pace. For example, if you're doing Paced Walking, start by walking at a deliberately slower pace, just to get your blood pumping. Or if you're doing slow jogging, jog in place. Two to three minutes at this slower pace should provide a sufficient warm-up.

Never neglect your warm-up! Sudden exertion without a gradual warm-up can lead to abnormal heart rate and inadequate blood flow to the heart, along with possible changes in blood pressure, all of which can be dangerous, particularly for older exercisers.

After you've finished exercising, be sure to cool down in order to allow your body time to readjust. Slow down gradually by decreasing the intensity of the activity to bring your body back to its resting state. Take an extra lap around the track, pedal the last five minutes slowly, or walk for five minutes after you've jogged.

Never stop suddenly after exercise. This can cause blood to pool in your muscles, reducing blood flow to your heart and brain. You could faint or experience abnormal rhythms in your heart—both of which could be dangerous.

Your Cardio Status: Special Guidelines for Special Situations

If you have already been exercising on a regular basis without any problems, by all means start out by exercising for 45 to 60 minutes. Other people may have to take it a little more slowly and not start the exercise portion of the program at full blastoff. Some of you need to take it slow and let your body gradually adapt to the new stress, particularly if you haven't exercised much in the past, if you're very overweight, or if you're advanced in age. There are several special conditions that may warrant tweaking your exercise prescription. If any of the following situations rings a bell with you, please don't take this lightly. Following these guidelines is vital to your overall health and well-being.

- *If you have a cardiovascular problem or any sort of health problem,* get your physician's blessing before you begin an exercise program. If you're approved, have your physician determine your Fat-Burning Zone and the level of intensity that is appropriate for you. Only then should you proceed.

- *If you are 100 pounds or more overweight,* consult with your physician before beginning this program. Find out medically what you can do to start. Many people who are overweight get winded just walking to the mailbox. Carrying extra pounds forces your heart and body to work overtime, and consequently you can reach your Fat-Burning Zone very quickly. Shoot for just 50 to 55 percent of your maximum heart rate and walk for at least five minutes. Slowly add a minute or two to that time, or as much as your body will comfortably allow. Keep adding minutes beyond the 12 days of this program so that you can begin to incorporate fat-burning exercise into your lifestyle.

- *If you are out of shape, are 50 pounds or more overweight, and/or are advanced in age,* start with 5 to 10 minutes of easy walking or stationary bicycling at 55 percent of your maximum heart rate (but get your doctor's okay first!). Slowly add to that time as your body becomes more accustomed to exercise. Continue to exercise beyond the 12 days of this program, gradually adding time to your routine, for optimum fat-burning effectiveness.

- *If you have done little or no cardiovascular exercise in the past, but are otherwise in good health,* start with only 10 to 15 minutes at 55 percent of your maximum as your Fat-Burning Zone. Add as many minutes as feels comfortable and doable to you. Beyond the 12 days of the program, work toward increasing your time to 45 minutes. Then slowly increase your prescribed heart rate in 5 percent increments until you reach 65 percent of your maximum. That way, you'll keep your body in a fat-burning mode each time you exercise.

- *If you are in reasonably good shape, and 50 pounds or less overweight,* start with 20 to 30 minutes at 60 percent of your maximum. Slowly add 5 to 10 minutes to your time as you are able and as you become aerobically more fit. Eventually, work your way up to 45 minutes to an hour per session. At the same time, shoot for increasing your intensity to 65 percent of your maximum in order to reach your Fat-Burning Zone.

Make It Fun

For long slow distance exercise to be maximally effective for fat loss over the next 12 days, you must do it four to even six times a week. But if you're like many people, you probably get bored to tears doing a repetitive activity for 45 minutes to an hour. Here are some pointers on how to avoid boredom while performing long slow distance exercise:

- Strap on headphones and use a lightweight portable stereo to listen to your favorite music, books on tape, or Body Makeover motivational audiotapes and CDs (see appendix B for information) while you're walking or jogging outdoors. Caution: Make sure you can still hear traffic noises. Ignoring what's going on around you can be risky.
- Watch television while pedaling on a stationary bicycle or walking on a treadmill. Or listen to music, motivational audiotapes, or CDs. If your equipment has a reading rack, read a book or a magazine.
- Change the scenery. If you get bored by your treadmill workout, take a walk outdoors instead.
- Vary your path. If you walk or jog outdoors on the same route every day, consider changing your path to alleviate the sameness.
- Find a makeover buddy. Recruit a friend or friends to do the *12-Day Body Shaping Miracle* with you—including the long slow distance exercise program. You can support each other, help each other when one of you wants to quit, and be inspired by each other's success and progress. Exercising with a buddy is motivating and provides the support you need to see the program through. Plus, it can make the next 12 days fun!

TO ACCELERATE FAT LOSS . . . AVOID THESE WORKOUTS!

Surprise: Some of the most popular workouts that are effective for cardiovascular fitness are not effective for burning fat. If you really want to burn fat, stick to long, slow, rhythmic workouts such as Paced Walking, slow jogging, a walk/jog, treadmill exercise, or stationary bicycling. Any exercise that has you working too strenuously burns sugar, not fat. A number of these are listed below.

Stair climbing

Elliptical machines

Aerobic dancing

Aerobic step classes

Kickboxing

Stair-step machines

Circuit training (with weights or machines)

Climbing machines (or vertical climbing walls)

Rowing machines

Martial arts

Boxing

Power cycling (Spinning-type classes)

Use long slow distance cardio to reveal your natural sexy curves. This one small change in your activity level adds up to big results—in terms of your fat burn, fitness, and endurance. By the end of the next 12 days, you'll clearly see why this form of exercise is worth the effort—and you'll be very proud of what you've accomplished and how great you look.

CHAPTER 8

My Figure-Shaping Nutrition Plan

exercise is one surefire way to take off pounds and change your shape, as long as you're watching your diet, too. In this chapter, I'll give you some meal-plan guidelines. But let me encourage you to look into two other sources that delve into my diet in more detail: the *6-Week Body Makeover* program, available from www.provida.com, or my book *6-Day Body Makeover*, an effective, short-term approach to dropping a pant or dress size in six days.

As in all of my makeover programs, the *12-Day Body Shaping Miracle* meal plans are customized to your body type. They include protein-source foods for muscle toning, carbohydrates for fuel, and fruits and vegetables to aid digestion, fight water retention, and deliver to your body significant amounts of health-building nutrients.

What you must eat while following this 12-day program is spelled out for you in step-by-step fashion. By the end of the 12 days, your clothes will feel less tight and you'll begin to look fabulous. With that in mind, let's get going. Here is my 10-point dietary strategy to help you change your shape—painlessly, without deprivation or starvation.

Point 1. Dine on Multiple Meals of Whole Foods

An important premise of my diet is eating five to six meals a day in order to keep you fueled and to keep your metabolism fired up for more efficient fat burning. Moreover, your meals should consist of whole foods—no processed foods. By *whole foods,* I mean those that are as close to nature as possible: vegetables, fruits, grains, and lean proteins. These types of foods are used more efficiently by your body, and they fill you up more completely but without being converted to body fat. Eating multiple meals of whole foods is an essential part of good weight control. Here is a closer look at why:

- *A higher metabolic rate.* Every time you eat a meal, your metabolic rate goes up as heat is given off to digest and absorb food. By eating five to six meals a day, your metabolism has extra opportunities to stay cranked up, and that means more fat-burning power.
- *More energy.* When you eat a balance of whole foods, including protein, unprocessed carbohydrates, low-sugar fruits, and low-starch vegetables, your food digests more slowly. This keeps your blood glucose levels steady for greater energy. With frequent meals, your body has a constant stream of energy-giving nutrients. When it's time to exercise, you'll be full of pep and ready to go.
- *Better absorption of nutrients.* Eating smaller, more frequent meals helps your body better use vitamins and minerals. Research has shown that a higher percentage of nutrients are absorbed with a series of small meals, compared with just two or three large ones.
- *Less temptation.* You'll be less inclined to stray from your fat-losing nutritional program. When you're eating five or six times a day, every two to three hours, you're less likely to binge on foods you shouldn't have. Nor will you get hungry or be prone to cravings. In short, frequent meals help tame hunger pangs and shore up your willpower.

Point 2. Eat According to Your Body Type

In addition to identifying your body shape, the Blueprint you took in chapter 2 is essential in determining how your body responds to different types of food. Not all metabolisms are created equal. Everyone is different. Not everyone can eat exactly the same foods the same way and get the same results. Foods that help one person stay lean may have no impact on another person, and someone else may gain weight eating those same foods. You must customize your diet to your own unique metabolism and biochemistry. When that happens, weight loss becomes automatic, because you've created a chemical reaction in your body with predictable results. *Make sure you have identified your body type before beginning your eating plan. Once you've done that, you can start your plan.*

Point 3. Stick to Permissible Foods

In the realm of body-shaping nutrition, you need a mix of lean proteins for muscular development and different types of natural carbohydrates for energy. You should also include plenty of green vegetables to prevent water retention (an enemy of a healthy metabolism), as well as other fruits and vegetables to supply numerous other health benefits. That said, let me review with you the best foods for body shaping and fat loss.

Lean Protein

Protein is to your body what a wood frame is to your house, or steel is to a bridge. Nutritionally, it is the basic, most important building material in your body, essential to high-level health because of its role in growth and maintenance.

The exercising body requires ample protein to develop and maintain body-firming muscle. In digestion, protein is broken down into subunits called *amino acids,* which are reshuffled back into protein to make and repair body tissues. Certain amino acids used in building muscle proteins can be burned by the body during exercise, especially intense aerobic workouts, so you want to make sure your protein intake is sufficient. This is one of the main reasons exercisers need a little more protein in their diets than sedentary people. If you don't get enough, your body can start breaking down muscle tissue to get amino acids for energy. Consequently, you'll lose metabolically active muscle and sabotage your body-shaping efforts.

Protein also keeps your immune system functioning up to par, helps carry nutrients throughout the body, has a hand in forming hormones, and is involved in important enzyme reactions such as digestion. My diet is purposely high in protein because it stimulates the reduction of body fat, particularly in the abdominal region, according to the latest research into dietary protein and fat loss.

Here is a rundown of the top protein choices, including which ones to eat for your body type:

• **Fish.** Your body will metabolize, or burn up, white fish such as sole or flounder more quickly than heavy red meat. Most people who need to drop body fat can experience rapid results with fish because it is metabolized very quickly and really stokes up the body's fat-burning furnace. If you don't like fish, of course, don't eat it. If a diet "forces" you to eat something you dislike, then you won't stay with that diet for very long. In place of fish, you can substitute skinless chicken or turkey breasts, or another lean protein choice.

Best for: All body types, especially A, B, and C, who tend to have the slowest metabolisms of all.

• **Chicken breast.** Lean chicken breast metabolizes rapidly, too. Make the right choices, however. Avoid rotisserie-cooked chicken from the supermarket, for example. It is generally loaded with both sodium and fat. Be careful, too, about buying big packages of frozen chicken breast meat. These products are often injected with high-sodium chicken broth or turkey broth to enhance the meat's flavor. Be sure to take the skin off your chicken breasts. Poultry skin is loaded with fat.

Best for: All body types.

• **Turkey breast.** This lean protein is abundant in protein for accentuating the muscle-toning process, and very low in fat compared with meats. For weight loss and general good health, you must limit the amount of fat you consume, and eating turkey breast is one way to do that. Dietary fat can cause weight gain and interferes with your metabolism. Be sure to eat skinless turkey breasts.

Best for: All body types.

• **Lean red meat.** Red meat contains iron, vitamin B$_{12}$, and certain amino acids that will help enhance lean muscle on your body. Another top-drawer nutrient in red meat is creatine, which is involved in building body-defining muscle. Creatine is also responsible for boosting the pace of energy production in your cells, so to some degree it helps you push harder and longer in workouts.

Caution: You'll need to choose the very leanest cuts of meat, because fat will slow your metabolism. These cuts include bottom round, eye of round, round tip (sirloin tip), tenderloin, top loin (strip loin), top round, and top sirloin.

Best for: Body Types D and E. One of the biggest problems for these body types is insufficient muscle. Any nutrient that will assist in toning and firming lean muscle (in partnership with exercise) will accelerate your metabolism, help you burn more fat, and assist in weight loss.

• **Egg whites.** These are the fastest-metabolizing proteins of all. Egg protein is commonly considered the "perfect protein" and is the common reference with which all other proteins are compared. You simply can't go wrong including egg whites in your diet. Most of the egg's protein is concentrated in the white, and egg whites contain virtually no fat, making them ideal for a body-shaping diet. Please note that egg whites are rather high in sodium, so if you are on a sodium-restricted diet, you may want to limit your intake, or substitute another lean protein.

Best for: All body types.

Low-Starch Vegetables

Eating more low-starch vegetables such as broccoli, cauliflower, asparagus, and greens can help enhance weight loss. These vegetables are high in fiber, too.

A growing body of research shows that high-fiber eating helps peel off pounds and banish them for good.

How exactly does fiber work this weight-loss magic?

Mainly by controlling your appetite. Because fibrous foods provide bulk, you feel full while eating a meal, so you're less tempted to overeat. High-fiber foods also take longer to chew, so your meals last longer. That's a plus, since it takes about 20 minutes after starting a meal for your body to send signals that it's full. When eaten with other nutrients such as protein, fiber slows the rate of digestion, too, keeping your energy levels steady throughout the day. Fiber slows your appetite between meals, makes you feel full, and keeps materials (including fat and calories) moving through your system at a healthy clip. Fiber also has the ability to bring down LDL cholesterol (the harmful type) and blood pressure.

Low-starch vegetables are among the best fuels to put in your body because they're so supercharged with vitamins, minerals, antioxidants, and phytochemicals to keep your immune system healthy, to help your body properly use the amino acids and complex carbs it's getting, and for optimum performance.

Broccoli and cauliflower, in particular, contain phytochemicals called indoles, which appear to help lower estrogen levels naturally in the body. Estrogen is a potentially fat-storing hormone.

If you've seen the diets I planned for participants on ABC's *Extreme Makeover*, you know that I loaded them with asparagus. This nutritious vegetable exerts a diuretic effect, allowing your body to lose water. Water retention interferes with your metabolism, so you want to fight it at every turn. Asparagus is also plentiful in an antioxidant called glutathione. Glutathione helps produce hormone-like messengers called prostaglandins, which, in turn, influence the development of lean, body-shaping muscle. Eat several servings of asparagus every week. Other great diuretic foods include greens and cucumbers. Increasing your intake of diuretic vegetables can further accelerate your metabolism.

Other highly desirable vegetables to add to your diet (in controlled portions) include alfalfa sprouts, bean sprouts, beet greens, bell peppers, dandelion greens, eggplant, endive, escarole, garlic, kale, leek, lettuce (all varieties), mushrooms (all varieties), mustard greens, okra, onion, radishes, shallots, spaghetti squash (makes a great substitute for pasta and noodles), spinach, string beans, summer squash, Swiss chard, tomatoes, turnip greens, watercress, and zucchini.

Low-Sugar Fruits

When you want to optimize your fat loss, it's best to stick to low-sugar fruits. Although fruits are extremely healthy, some do call forth the hormone insulin to handle the sugars they contain. Insulin is another potentially fat-forming hormone, so you want to keep your insulin regulated as much as possible during fat loss. The fiber content of these fruits will make you feel full, too. Fruit juices are always too high in sugars to fit with a body-shaping style of eating, so forgo juices while losing fat.

The following fruits are your best choices during fat loss because they are low in sugar: apples (Granny Smith apples especially), blackberries, blueberries, boysenberries, cantaloupe, cherries, elderberries, gooseberries, grapefruit, honeydew melon, lemons and limes, peaches, pears, plums, raspberries, strawberries, and tangerines.

Complex Carbohydrates

Complex carbohydrates such as beans, rice, potatoes, yams, and legumes are terrific energy foods, and you need them in your diet. They are required to make and replenish muscle glycogen, the carbohydrate stored in the muscles and liver and used to supply energy for exercise and activity. Carbohydrates also supply that amazing fat-fighting nutrient—fiber.

Complex carbs contain two types of fiber: soluble and insoluble. Found in oats, barley, and beans, soluble fiber helps lower cholesterol. Oats, fruits, and vegetables are food sources of insoluble fiber, which keeps your digestive tract healthy and free from cancer-causing substances. Oats and barley, in particular, have been shown in research to reduce glucose and insulin responses and the risk of obesity.

Avoid processed carbohydrates such as refined pasta and bread products which are less effective in a fat-loss program. These foods have undergone too much processing and consequently are not utilized as well, with more of a tendency to be converted into body fat. Shun these foods while you're losing fat, and you'll notice a huge difference in your body definition and shape.

The complex carbs I recommend include barley, jicama, millet, oatmeal, oat bran, parsnips, potato, rutabagas, squash (winter), sweet potatoes, turnips, and rice (brown rice, long-grain rice, and wild rice are best).

Point 4. Eliminate Fast Carbs

Simple carbs and sugars—honey, syrup, table sugar, brown sugar, candy, sugary desserts, sweets, all processed carbs—are quickly digested into glucose, a sugar in the blood that is converted into glycogen for the muscles and liver or carried in the blood to fuel the brain and muscles. I refer to these foods as fast carbs because they are transformed to sugar very quickly by your body. This category includes sweet foods such as sugary desserts, cakes, cookies, fruit juice, sugared sodas, certain types of sweet fruits, and all processed carbs (bread, bread products, pasta, sugared cereals, and so forth).

If you eat too many fast carbs, they can be turned into body fat. This happens because their excessive sugar content triggers a surge of the hormone insulin. Insulin activates certain enzymes that promote fat storage. Natural, complex carbohydrates don't cause this reaction—which is why they're less likely to be stored as fat. So avoid fast carbs when you're losing body fat.

If you're among the many people who have trouble losing body fat because of sweets, take heart. Yes, we're genetically programmed to love the taste of sugar from the moment we're born. But you can wean yourself away from fast carbs and sweets. Generally, it takes about five to seven days. Afterward, your taste buds will change so dramatically that you won't even need that sugar fix. However, if you get hypoglycemic (low blood sugar), you may need a fast carb.

Point 5. Slash Fat Calories

Fatty foods can fast derail your attempts to shape up. The main reason: Calories from fat (butter, fried foods, cheeses, candy, and so forth) are readily stored as body fat, whereas calories from other foods have to be converted to fat—a process that burns calories. For ongoing fat loss, eliminate fatty foods that could slow or halt your progress altogether. These include:

Oils, especially tropical, saturated types
Butter, margarine, shortening, lard
Nuts and nut butters
Dairy, including milk, sour cream, any kind of cheese, and ice cream
Processed foods, including commercially baked foods and deli meat
Salad dressings and mayonnaise
Fatty cuts of meat
Vegetable oil sprays

Be especially careful to shun *trans fats,* synthetic fats created through the refining of healthy oils. These fats are found in most fried foods and commercially baked goods; the red flag on the ingredients list is "partially hydrogenated vegetable oil." Your body has a difficult time burning these fats, so stay away from this gunk if you're serious about losing weight.

Point 6. Serve Up Controlled Portions

For the *12-Day Body Shaping Miracle* to work effectively, you must pay strict attention to your portions—the amount of protein, carbohydrates, vegetables, greens, and fruits you eat at each meal. This is important, since certain nutrients are not assimilated or converted into fuel when eaten in excess amounts, wreaking havoc on your metabolism. A nutritious diet includes the right servings and portions of the following foods every day, depending on your body type:

• Two to three servings of fresh fruit and three or more servings of vegetables, depending on your body type. Examples of a serving: a medium piece of fruit, or 1 to 2 cups of vegetables.

- Two to three servings of natural complex carbohydrates, depending on your body type: ½ cup cooked rice, half a medium baked potato or sweet potato, and ½ cup cooked beans or legumes.
- Several servings of protein-rich foods: 2 ounces of white meat chicken, fish, or lean red meat, or two to three egg whites.

The best way to control your portions is to weigh and measure your food—after cooking it. But if weighing and measuring isn't practical for you, you'll find in the following chart some instructions for estimating portion sizes with foods common to this program. Weigh and measure your foods after cooking them to get the right amounts, since most foods shrink after being cooked.

Food	Portion Size
Protein (fish, poultry breast, or lean meat)	2 ounces = a small packet of matches, or a tea bag
Carbohydrates	½ cup rice = your hand when cupped; 1 cup rice = your fist; 1 medium potato, sweet potato, or yam = tennis ball
Vegetables and greens	1 cup = your fist
Fruits	1 piece = baseball; ½ cup berries = your hand when cupped

Point 7. De-emphasize Sodium for Accelerated Weight Loss

Here is something that may surprise you: One of the unrecognized keys to fast yet safe weight loss is to control the amount of sodium you consume. You know sodium best as table salt, but salt and sodium are hidden in all kinds of products, including packaged foods, fast foods, sodas, frozen and canned foods, condiments, and other food products. No matter where it hides out, excess sodium in your diet will dramatically slow your metabolism.

How is this possible? The answer is water retention. When you eat more salt than you need, some of the extra sodium is deposited just beneath your skin. There it attracts water, which is retained in your cells. This watery logjam not only adds pounds, but also distorts the shape of your body and keeps you from getting even your "fat" clothes to fit. You look and feel puffy, miserable, and uncomfortable, because it feels like you've gained 10 pounds or more.

As your body metabolizes, or burns fat, the by-product is water. To make the fat-burning process as efficient as possible, your body requires a steady flow of fluid in and out of your body. If water gets dammed up in your cells, this flow is obstructed, thus making you bloated. Think of it this way: Slowing the flow out is like putting a potato in the tailpipe of your car; it dramatically reduces the efficiency of the engine. Similarly, sodium-induced water retention has the potential to dramatically slow or stop your body's engine—your metabolism.

While this may sound disheartening, there is one simple way to get rid of the cause of bloating and impaired metabolism: Put down the saltshaker and avoid foods containing a lot of sodium! While following this program, you must totally eliminate salt from your diet, unless you have low blood pressure. You need salt if you have been diagnosed with low blood pressure. Most people, however, need to trade in processed foods for fresh, homemade versions. Precooked meats, lunch meats, and packaged foods are loaded with sodium.

True, salt is an important source of sodium and iodine. Sodium works together with potassium, another required mineral, to assist nerve stimulation and regulate water balance. It is also involved in carbohydrate absorption. And yes, we need some sodium in our diets, but most people eat too much. Your body needs only 500 milligrams of sodium daily for good health, and you can obtain this amount through your diet, without additional salt. For perspective, if you have been in the habit of salting your foods, keep in mind that each shake of your saltshaker provides about 100 milligrams of sodium.

Salt is present naturally in just about every type of food. So if you eat a normal amount of healthy food, you'll almost certainly get all the salt you need. But what if you have a "salt tooth"? Don't worry: Once you start cutting down on salt, you'll lose your taste for it.

In addition, controlling salt intake is an important health measure if you are suffering from high blood pressure. So instead of salt, experiment with herbs and nonsodium seasonings to enhance the flavor of your meals. Read labels carefully, too. Many fast foods are loaded with sodium.

If you have low blood pressure (90/60 or lower), however, you may carry salt with you because you need it. So in your case, salt your food.

Point 8. Pump the Water

Your primary beverage should be water—in the amount of 12 full 8-ounce glasses a day, or approximately 100 ounces—while following the *12-Day Body Shaping Miracle*. This is a simple secret that will accelerate your fat loss.

I know what you're probably saying: "Michael, that's a lot of water! I can't drink that much!" But hear me out on this: Drinking more water can actually help reduce body fat. Here is the reason why: Your kidneys rely on water to do their job of filtering waste products and impurities from your body. With a water shortage, the kidneys cannot function properly, so they dump their workload on the liver. Among the liver's many functions is to metabolize stored fat into usable fuel for your body. But if your liver has to take on an extra assignment from the kidneys, its ability to burn fat is severely compromised. If less fat is metabolized, more of it remains stored, and weight loss stops. You must drink enough water to help your body metabolize stored fat.

Drinking enough water each day also helps prevent fluid retention. When your body gets less water than it requires, it perceives this shortage as a threat to survival and will start hoarding water. This survival response shows up in swollen feet, hands, and legs, and an overall distorted body shape and extra poundage in the form of retained water. Remember, fluid retention interferes with metabolism.

Point 9. Be Wary of Condiments

Lurking in many condiments are sugar and salt—two bulge makers our diets can do without. Condiments are one of the quickest ways to gain weight! Try enjoying the true taste of fresh food without condiments. Do whatever you need to do, within the parameters of your eating plan, to make your food enjoyable. Try herbs and spices to excite your taste buds and break the monotony. Don't forget the role your eyes play in making food palatable, either. A plate of white meat chicken, white cauliflower, and a white potato can be boring to your eyes. So try making your meals as colorful as possible to delight not only your eyes but your taste buds, too.

Point 10. Avoid All Alcoholic Beverages, Including Nonalcoholic Beers and Wines, as Well as Juice

These beverages are all very high in calories and simple sugars and have the ability to slow down your metabolism and dramatically reduce weight loss. What most people don't understand is that alcohol is metabolized in the body like a sugar. That means it ends up being stored as body fat. Alcohol is high in simple sugars, which will slow the weight-loss process. If you want to be successful on this program, you must give up alcohol while losing weight and changing your shape.

Fruit juices are full of sugar. It may take 10 oranges to make a glass of orange juice, and that translates into lots of sugar. Sugar—even that from fruit juice—spikes insulin. If you are experiencing low blood sugar, however, I certainly recommend fruit juice to help get your blood sugar back on an even keel. Just don't use it as a daily staple when you're trying to lose weight.

REMINDERS

- Do not deviate from the permissible foods that were listed previously or are listed in your menus.
- Follow your eating plan exactly as specified. *Make no substitutions* (unless you're substituting lean poultry for fish).
- Pay strict attention to portion sizes.
- Do not use oil, mayonnaise, commercial salad dressings, butter, margarine, vegetable oil spray, or any other added oils or fats.
- Never skip any meals, except for your optional PM snack.
- Drink 12 full 8-ounce glasses of water daily.

Following My Figure-Shaping Plan

Each customized menu plan below lists for you exactly what to eat throughout the day: lean proteins, natural complex carbohydrates, low-starch vegetables, greens, and low-sugar fruits. If a food isn't on your list, don't eat it!

To start seeing results, you must eat every meal (each spaced between two and three hours apart), and you must eat the meals in the prescribed order. Please do not transpose meals or you might significantly disrupt the intended goal of keeping your metabolism in fat-burning mode.

Here are some important notes on medical conditions: The way to completely customize your diet is to refer to the numbers of your blood pressure reading. If it's high—such as 90 on the bottom and 140 to 150 on the top—eliminate salt or sodium. But do so in consultation with your physician. If your blood pressure is low, say 60 on the bottom and 100 (or below) on the top, you will need to add salt to your diet.

If you typically cannot go for a long period of time without eating, you must add a carbohydrate to each meal. Not being able to go without food for more than three to four hours can be a sign of low blood sugar. Good choices for additional carbs include fruits such as pineapple, cantaloupe, or grapefruit; these make great between-meal snacks. (If you're taking prescription medicines, find out whether grapefruit will cause any interfering reactions.) Also, if you have low blood sugar, you may need a carb with each meal.

If you have diabetes, you may have to cut carbs from certain meals, with the exception of pre-exercise meals. Or you may have to remove the carbs from meals when your blood sugar is high. It is very important if you are a diabetic to monitor your blood sugar levels and to work with your physician concerning your diet. Diabetes really requires your physician's help in order to properly customize your diet.

Take this book to your physician and have him or her help you customize it accordingly. Everyone is different, and body type is not the sole criterion for customization. Work with your physician concerning your individual needs. For more information on customizing for special medical conditions, refer to appendix A.

SAMPLE EATING PLANS FOR YOUR BODY TYPE

BODY TYPE A ENDO	BODY TYPE B ENDO-MESO	BODY TYPE C MESO-ENDO	*BODY TYPE D ENDO-ECTO	*BODY TYPE E ECTO-ENDO
Breakfast: 2 egg whites, or 2 oz. turkey breast; 1 serving oatmeal, millet, or brown rice; and 1 serving fruit	*Breakfast:* 2 egg whites, or 2 oz. turkey breast; 1 serving oatmeal, millet, or brown rice; and 1 serving fruit	*Breakfast:* 2 egg whites, or 2 oz. turkey breast; 1 serving oatmeal, millet, or brown rice; and 1 serving fruit	*Breakfast:* 2 oz. lean beef and 2–3 egg whites; 1 serving oatmeal, millet, or brown rice; and 1 serving fruit	*Breakfast:* 2 oz. lean beef and 2–3 egg whites; 1 serving oatmeal, millet, or brown rice; and 1 serving fruit
Midmorning snack: 2 oz. protein and 1 cup greens	*Midmorning snack:* 2 oz. turkey breast and 1 cup greens	*Midmorning snack:* 2 oz. protein and 1–2 cups greens	*Midmorning snack:* 2 oz. lean beef and 1 cup greens	*Midmorning snack:* 2 oz. lean beef and 1–2 cups greens
Lunch: 2 oz. protein, ½ medium potato or yam or other allowed complex carb, and 1 cup greens	*Lunch:* 2 oz. chicken breast, ½ cup brown rice or other allowed complex carb, and 1 cup mixed vegetables	*Lunch:* 2 oz. chicken breast, ½ cup brown rice or other allowed complex carb, and 1–2 cups mixed vegetables	*Lunch:* 2 oz. chicken breast, ½ cup brown rice or other allowed complex carb, and 1 cup mixed vegetables	*Lunch:* 2 oz. chicken breast, ½ cup brown rice or ½ cup beans and brown rice (combined to make ½ cup), and 1–2 cups mixed vegetables
Midafternoon snack: 2 oz. protein and 1 cup greens	*Midafternoon snack:* 2 oz. fish and 1 cup greens	*Midafternoon snack:* 2 oz. fish and 1 cup greens	*Midafternoon snack:* 2 oz. chicken breast and 1 cup greens	*Midafternoon snack:* 2 oz. lean beef and 1 serving fruit
Dinner: 2 oz. protein, ½ medium potato or yam or other allowed complex carb, and 1 cup greens	*Dinner:* 2 oz. chicken breast, ½ cup brown rice or other allowed complex carb, and 1 cup mixed vegetables	*Dinner:* 2 oz. chicken breast, ½ cup brown rice or other allowed complex carb, and 1–2 cups mixed vegetables	*Dinner:* 2 oz. chicken breast, ½ cup brown rice or other allowed complex carb, and 1 cup mixed vegetables	*Dinner:* 2 oz. chicken breast, ½ cup brown rice or ½ cup beans and brown rice (combined to make ½ cup) and 1–2 cups mixed vegetables
Optional PM snack: 2 oz. chicken breast and 1 cup greens	*Optional PM snack:* 1 serving fruit	*Optional PM snack:* 1 serving fruit	*Optional PM snack:* 2 oz. protein and 1 cup greens or mixed vegetables	*Optional PM snack:* 2 oz. chicken breast and 1 serving fruit

* If you are a Body Type D or E, bump up your protein serving to 3 ounces at meals eaten after your workout. Slightly increasing your protein during these times assists in the development of lean, curvaceous muscle.

Pre-Prepare Meals for Ease and Convenience

You eat a lot of food on this plan, and if you're as busy as most people, it's not always easy to get motivated to make meals. You're probably wondering, *How do I find time to cook and fix all this food?* The answer is amazingly simple: Shop once a week from a shopping list and cook your meals ahead of time, in bulk. Think of it this way: It doesn't take any longer to cook four chicken breasts than it does to cook one.

Here are some suggestions for pre-preparing your food that will make meal planning a cinch:

- Hard-boil your eggs, store them in the refrigerator, and you'll have egg whites ready to go. Or break fresh eggs, eliminate the yolk, place the whites in a plastic container with a small amount of water, microwave, add pepper, and your breakfast is ready.
- Preslice your fruit and store it in a plastic container in the refrigerator until you're ready to eat it.
- Buy "salad in a bag"—lettuce and greens that are precut for convenience.
- Steam and store your vegetables in the refrigerator; they'll keep for two to three days without losing their freshness. To reheat steamed veggies, add a bit of water and microwave in a bowl for a few seconds. They'll taste like they've been freshly steamed.
- Bake, microwave, or boil potatoes or sweet potatoes by the dozen. They will keep for a week in your refrigerator as long as they are sealed in a container. To reheat them, simply pop them in the microwave for a minute or less.
- Boil rice ahead of time and store it in the refrigerator. It will keep for two to three days before spoiling. Or try the Japanese sticky-style rice; it stays moist and usable longer than other varieties.
- Bake a turkey breast, cover it with a wet paper towel to preserve moisture, and store it in the refrigerator. Reheat your portion in the microwave when you need it for a meal.

- Marinate and grill a dozen chicken breasts on the barbecue, then store them in a plastic container in the refrigerator. When you're ready to eat, pop them in the microwave with a little marinade sauce, and you've got protein anytime. Do the same for lean beef if it's on your custom eating plan.
- Store fish frozen. Season and cook the amount of fish you need for the next days. Then cut it into right-sized portions and wrap the pieces in individual plastic packets. Put all the packets in a freezer bag to ensure freshness, and reheat in the microwave when needed. Also, buy plenty of small cans of no-sodium-added water-packed tuna to have on hand in a pinch.

Pre-Exercise Nutrition

The foods you're eating on the *12-Day Body Shaping Miracle* are meant not only to trigger weight loss, but also to energize your body for exercise. On the days that you perform your long slow distance cardio, *you must eat one of your allotted carbohydrates and protein (2-ounce portion) 30 minutes prior to exercising.* This combination helps fuel you for your workout. Eating a carbohydrate and a protein before exercising can make a huge difference in your energy levels and in your performance during a workout. To push through your workout, try to never skip your pre-exercise meal. Here's how to make that happen:

- If you're a Body Type A, eat 2 ounces of lean protein, and a baked potato or yam; or ½ cup of oatmeal plus a banana prior to exercising.
- If you're a Body Type B, eat 2 ounces of lean protein, cooked brown rice (in your serving size), and a banana; or a yam prior to exercising.
- If you're a Body Type C, eat 2 ounces of lean protein, cooked brown rice (in your serving size), and a banana prior to exercising.
- If you're a Body Type D, eat 2 ounces of lean protein, cooked brown rice (in your serving size), and a banana prior to exercising.
- If you're a Body Type E, eat 2 ounces of lean protein, and cooked brown rice or beans (in your serving size); or ½ cup of oatmeal and a banana prior to exercising.

Post-Exercise Nutrition

In the wake of a workout, a process called recovery takes place in your body. To appreciate its importance, consider what happens inside your body as a consequence of exercising: Energy-giving glycogen stores are depleted; muscle protein is dismantled; microscopic tears in muscle fibers occur; energy-producing compounds are lost from cells; and fluids and electrolytes (minerals) dwindle.

To restore what has been depleted, you've got to supply it with all the nutritional building blocks it needs to replace what's lost and repair what's damaged. The benefits of doing this are numerous: greater energy levels each time you work out, less fatigue, and better muscular development (which enhances your emerging, sexy curves).

Of all the nutrients necessary for optimum recovery, dietary carbohydrate takes precedence for two reasons. First, carbohydrate restocks your body with glycogen, which can be depleted during exercise. Replenishing these stores allows you to exercise more energetically on successive workouts for better gains. Second, carbohydrate prevents muscle from being broken down to provide energy for resistance exercise; in other words, it helps spare muscle.

When you add protein to your post-exercise carb meal, the net effect is to create a hormonal environment in your body that enhances the development of lean, attractive muscle. This nutrient combination also jump-starts your body's glycogen-making process—faster than if you consumed carbs alone. Why such speed? Carbs produce a positive surge in insulin levels. Biochemically, insulin is like an accelerator pedal that races the body's glycogen-utilizing motor.

Following your workout, schedule one of your morning or afternoon snacks, as follows:

- If you're a Body Type A, eat 2 ounces of lean protein. As your carbohydrate, eat a baked potato, yam, or brown rice; or an apple, peach, or pear.
- If you're a Body Type B, eat 2 ounces of lean protein. As your carbohydrate, eat a baked potato, yam, or brown rice; or an apple, peach, or pear.

- If you're a Body Type C, eat 2 ounces of lean protein. As your carbohydrate, eat a baked potato, yam, or brown rice; or an apple, peach, or pear.
- If you're a Body Type D, eat 3 ounces of lean protein. As your carbohydrate, eat a baked potato, yam, or brown rice; or an apple, peach, or pear.
- If you're a Body Type E, eat 3 ounces of lean protein. As your carbohydrate, eat a baked potato, yam, or brown rice; or an apple, peach, or pear.

Make the Commitment

Because you're beginning to change your shape in just 12 days, there is little room for deviation from this program. After getting approval from your physician, please commit to every nutritional point covered here without fail.

Do yourself and your body a favor: Approach these 12 days with a can-do attitude—and you will begin to see your newly resculpted body before too long!

Beyond the First 12 Days: Look Better than Ever, Forever

Now that you've begun to change your shape and are seeing an attractive, noticeable transformation in your mirror, it's time to think about continuing your progress and ultimately maintaining your new shape. The momentum you have built over the last 12 days should be like a jet-propulsion force, giving you tremendous impetus to achieve even greater body-shaping success. At this point, you ought to be even more highly motivated and highly intentioned. That said, what should you be doing now that you've completed the 12-day program?

If you like what you see in the mirror and if you like how you feel, you can repeat the program for another 12 days. Or you may wish to try my *6-Week Body Makeover* if you need more time to redesign your body. What I ultimately want for you is a total lifestyle change so that you can maintain your hot new body and stay healthy for a lifetime. This program is really about long-term success, not gimmicks. There's a reason why so many people quit exercising or eating right after only a few weeks or gain back the weight (with interest) after doing a gimmicky program. Most of these programs never talk about changing your lifestyle. A successful eating or workout plan also needs to look at whether it's something you can do for a lifetime. This chapter will give you important guidance to help you change your behavior, stay on the right path, and maintain the body you've always wanted—for a lifetime.

They Did It—and So Can You!

Before I get into the nuts and bolts of what to do beyond the next 12 days, let me share with you some additional success stories of women who started their transformation with the *12-Day Body Shaping Miracle* program and continued on to further sculpt their dream body beyond those initial but all-important 12 days. I hope you're inspired by their before-and-after photos. Here is what they have to say.

Natalya R., age 20

Went from a size 6 to a size 2 in two weeks!

I gained "the freshman 15" when I went away to college. Now thanks to Michael Thurmond, I don't have to worry about going back to school chunky. I lost 10 pounds and 13½ inches in just two weeks and I have so much energy now. This was easy! I can't wait to put a bikini on and show my friends how great I look on the beach!—*Natalya R.*

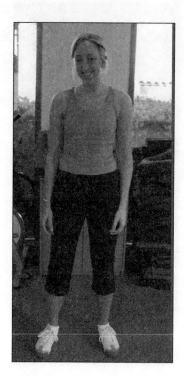

before

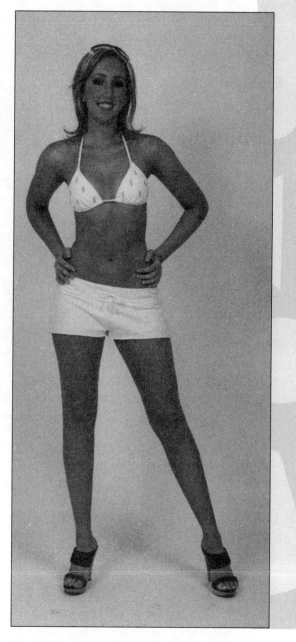

after

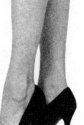

Szuszanna O., age 34
Went from a size 10 to a size 4 in three weeks!

After my baby, I couldn't get back into shape. I made the commitment to call Michael Thurmond, and it was the best call I ever made! I lost 25 inches in three weeks! I feel like a new person and look forward to keeping up with my toddler.—*Szuszanna O.*

after

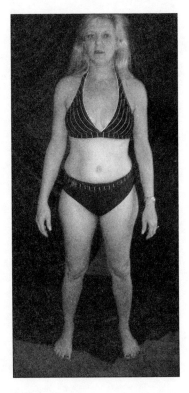

before

Bea D., age 50

Went from a size 10 to a size 8 in just six weeks!

I first saw Michael Thurmond on TV and thought his program sounded fantastic. Believe me; I have tried every diet and fat burning pills that are out there. I also had knee surgery eight years ago and, according to my doctor, was limited to what I could do. The results I saw within the first two weeks were amazing. And, after six weeks I had lost over 10 pounds, I'd lost inches from my chest, waist, and hips, and put on muscle density. This is my new lifestyle that I will continue.—*Bea*

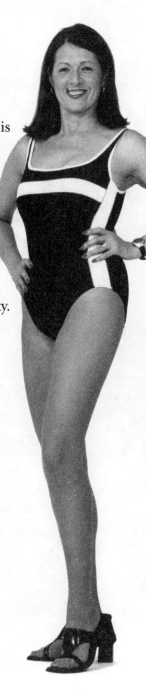

after

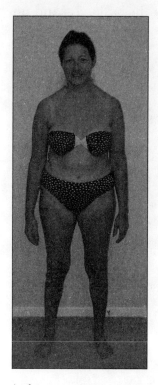

before

Carly A., age 23

Went from a size 12 to a size 7 in just six weeks!

I lost 20 pounds and 14 inches in just six weeks! Before coming to the Michael Thurmond Makeover program, losing weight on my own was becoming increasingly more frustrating! I really began to believe that my body was incapable of losing the weight that I gained in college. However, after my first week on Michael Thurmond's program I noticed a huge difference. After six weeks, I was not only thrilled about the 20 pounds I lost, but also the healthy and active lifestyle I gained. Thanks to Michael, I lost 4 inches from my waist, hips, and chest! I really feel that my main focus has shifted off what the scale says and on to how great I feel to be active again. Thank you, Body Makeovers!—*Carly*

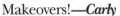

after

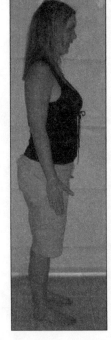

before

Create a Longer-Term Strategy with Realistic Goals

No doubt, you'll want to experience the same success these women did. After the initial 12 days, you may still want to tweak your figure in order to obtain your dream body. Maybe you have some more weight to lose, or perhaps you still want to work on specific parts of your body, such as lifting your buns, shrinking your thighs, or giving other parts of your body more overall tone. Whatever it is you want to change about your body, you can do it by using the techniques and methods you've been introduced to here. I can't say it too many times, or in too many different ways: You can do it! That's precisely where goal setting comes in—to make sure that you continue to do what it takes to create your ideal body.

People who are successful at developing their dream bodies have detailed goal-setting plans in place, including what they want to accomplish in the long term, as well as what they want to accomplish on a weekly or daily basis (again, what I refer to as mini-goals). It's a good idea to express your long-term goals in terms of an end result, such as improving your symmetry, losing weight, lowering your blood pressure, or having more energy. A goal like this must be realistic and attainable, with a time frame wrapped around it, or else it will be too vague. Choosing goals that are attainable with a definite period of time increases the probability that you will achieve them. If you want to lose 10, 20, even 30 pounds, for example, this is the kind of goal you can expect to achieve in as little as six weeks.

Your mini-goals from here on out should be process-oriented. By that, I mean they should describe the steps you'll take daily or weekly to meet your long-term goals. These steps are specific behaviors that will lead you to achieving those goals. Unless you come up with specific behaviors that are different from what you're doing now, you will have trouble obtaining your dream body. Examples of mini-goals might include jogging or walking four to five times a week, increasing the challenge (resistances) of your body-shaping routine each week, having a piece of fruit as an afternoon snack instead of a candy bar, making healthier choices at the grocery store, or following your food plan on a day-to-day basis. With realistic, attainable long-term goals and mini-goals, you can get further down the path of creating your dream body. Not only that, but the attainment of these goals is also associated with positive psychological changes such as greater self-confidence and motivation. You can think of your long-term goals as the top of a flight of stairs, whereas your mini-goals represent each step that will take you there.

To use goal setting to stay on track, first ask yourself what you want to achieve, say, over the next two to three months. Weight loss? A flatter stomach? Improved posture? A more defined body, overall? All of the above? The answers to this question form your long-term goals. If you are like most people, you probably have several long-term goals.

The next step is to define specific behaviors that you can do on a weekly and daily basis to reach your long-term goals. Remember, these are called mini-goals.

Then create a Goal-Setting Sheet like the one below on which you record all your goals. Writing down your goals drives home the need to achieve them.

GOAL-SETTING SHEET

My long-term goals (with a specific time line attached): (Example: Lose 15 pounds in six weeks)

My mini-goals (for each long-term goal, list the daily or weekly steps it will take to achieve it; it's a good idea to list your mini-goals for each day of the week):

Monday: _____

Tuesday: _____

Wednesday: _____

Thursday: _____

Friday: _____

Saturday: _____

Sunday: _____

More than 5,000 people to date have volunteered to participate in a university-based research study called the National Weight Control Registry. The participants have lost 66 pounds on average, and have kept it off for long periods of time. They're being studied to see how they did it. So far, this landmark study has revealed many characteristics common to successful weight maintenance:

- Eating a low-fat diet.
- Eating breakfast almost every day.
- Self-monitoring (for instance, weighing themselves frequently and keeping a food journal—as long as 20 years after weight loss)
- Engaging in physical activity for an hour each day (a majority chose walking).
- Eating five times a day.
- Eating out only periodically, but avoiding fast-food restaurants.

Unless you have goals in place, you may join the ever-swelling ranks of people who have reverted to their former out-of-shape bodies. It is an unfortunate fact that most dieters, in particular, can regain as much as two-thirds of their lost pounds within a year, and reacquire all of it within five years, according to the American Society of Bariatric Physicians (ASBP). You have come so far in only 12 short days, and I know you don't want to backslide!

Never stop rewarding yourself, either. Celebrate every accomplishment of your goals along the way. Give yourself something non-food-related. Maybe it's a new outfit, pampering at a day spa, a massage, new workout gear, or a new hairstyle—something that further fuels your motivation to look the best you can look. Create a nonfood reward list and use it every time you reach a goal.

Actively Pursue Your Dream Body

In addition to your diet, the most effective tool for creating your dream body is regular exercise, using the techniques and methods I have covered in this book.

Not only does exercise burn energy (calories) and keep your metabolism running in high gear, but it also enhances your self-image—how you feel about yourself. I hope as you experienced positive changes in your figure during these 12 days, you began to feel better about your body and your appearance, both of which contribute to your self-image in a big way. Over the long haul, a strong self-image is vital to weight maintenance, and research bears this out. People who frequently relapse, regaining their weight in the process, have very weak self-images. They see themselves as heavy or ugly and are generally dissatisfied with their bodies. Consequently, they do not have the psychological staying power to transform their bodies and their health.

The point is, you can continue to use the techniques, tools, and methods in this book to prop up your self-image, and in doing so stay the course toward creating your dream body.

As you go forward, be sure to keep your body-shaping workouts challenging. This involves coaxing your muscles to work a little harder each time you exercise. You can do this by progressively increasing your resistance, doing more repetitions, performing more sets, or all of these. Muscles adapt very quickly to stresses placed on them, so you'll want to give them new challenges to maximize your progress. Increasing your effort each workout makes your muscles get firmer, stronger, and shapelier. But don't forget to rest! If you feel tired, do not exercise until your body feels more energetic—a sign that it is demanding its workout. If at some point you take a layoff from exercising, start back slowly, lightly, and easily—in order to prevent injuries. Nor do you ever want to train a sore muscle. Let it recover with rest and proper nutrition, or else your body can break down and you'll exhaust yourself.

Generally, to add fullness to certain body parts, you'll want to increase your resistance while keeping your repetitions in the 8-to-12 range. The resistance must be enough to stimulate the muscles, yet not so much that you start using sloppy form. Use a resistance that lets you train in a good style, but is challenging enough to tax your muscles. More repetitions (12 or more) with lighter resistances lengthen your muscles and help make certain body parts appear more lean and slender.

As for your long slow distance cardio, there are two vital components to work

THINKING ABOUT SKIPPING YOUR WORKOUT? THINK AGAIN!

Anytime you're thinking about skipping your exercise session, whip out this list and remind yourself of what can happen if you stop exercising regularly:

- Muscles decrease in size, tone, and strength, and you'll begin to lose your desired body shape.
- The activity of fat-burning enzymes declines.
- Your muscles lose their ability to store energy-yielding glycogen.
- Your heart becomes deconditioned, and your body's aerobic power declines.
- You lose speed and flexibility.
- Body fat gradually returns, and fat cells enlarge.

on to increase your challenge: frequency and duration (time). If you still need to shed some body fat—and do it rather quickly—then you'll want to increase the frequency of your cardio, maybe to five or six times a week, if you're not already doing so. But if you can get it in only three times a week, not to worry. That's 100 percent better than doing nothing at all. The key is to keep performing your long slow distance cardio so that it becomes an ingrained lifestyle habit.

As for duration, try to gradually increase the length of time of your cardio. If you've been doing 30 minutes, increase your duration to 45 minutes; if you've been doing 45 minutes, increase your time to 60 minutes. Longer sessions, exercising at a lower intensity, can help you burn the most fat. If you started this program as a beginner, you probably worked out at a steady, comfortable pace. After a couple of weeks, take your intensity up a notch, while keeping it in your Fat-Burning Zone. You should always feel like your body is being challenged.

Keep an Eye on You

One of the truly successful techniques you can use to stay on track toward your body-shaping goals is self-monitoring, in which you keep close tabs on what you eat, your activity, your weight, and your measurements—even to the point of recording this information in a notebook or journal. Self-monitoring is actually an accountability system that helps you know where you are at any given time. Because it is difficult to refute what you've put down in print, a written record helps keep you honest about your habits and allows you to measure and evaluate your progress, then course-correct if necessary. There are several ways you can self-monitor, all of them important. For example:

• *Keep a food diary of what you eat each day, or plan to eat.* This doesn't mean recording every little fat gram or doing calorie counts—just staying conscious of the foods you're eating. A food diary can positively affect your eating behavior by helping you become more aware of your food choices. If you find yourself gaining weight, you can then adjust your eating accordingly.

• *Track your exercise progress in a training log.* Make it a point to write down when you exercised, how long you exercised, and if you increased the intensity or resistance of certain exercises. Writing down how many reps and sets you do in your workout, or keeping track of the frequency and duration of your cardio, can create motivating reminders of how much stronger, shapelier, and more aerobically fit you're becoming.

• *Step on the scale.* Is your weight climbing or declining? Because the scale doesn't lie, it saves you from self-deception and tells you whether you need to tighten up your eating habits, exercise more, or both. Research tells us that people who maintain their weight losses frequently monitor their weight in this fashion. In fact, many people weigh themselves as much as once a day; this, however, can lead to obsessive-compulsive behavior and is inaccurate anyway, since the body may gain fluid one day and lose it the next. I recommend weighing yourself once a week or every six days.

• *Check how your clothes fit.* I always advise that you wear clothing that fits you somewhat tightly (as opposed to baggy outfits) so that you are always aware of your body and tuned in to whether you are regaining any weight. If an article of clothing starts to feel too tight, that's a signal for you to get back on the weight-loss track. Monitoring yourself by using the scale and being aware of your clothes give you conscious control over the management of your weight. Measure yourself periodically, too. Always watch for changes in your weight and measurements, or in how your clothes fit, and respond to these changes quickly. Identify possible explanations for any changes in your weight:

Is it because of changes in your eating (too many sugary foods or high-fat foods, too much eating out, emotional overeating, increases in portion sizes, excessive alcohol intake, and so on)?

Is it due to a change in activity (fewer exercise sessions, not enough cardio, dropped out of exercising altogether)?

Could health issues or medication be contributing factors? (If so, please consult your physician.)

If you have slipped, climb back on that horse the very next meal and the very next workout. The only serious mistake you can make is to give up on your effort to change your body. When you backslide, which is normal, don't make excuses, either. Don't blame your metabolism. Don't blame your mom for pushing food at you. Don't blame your genes or anything else you think is beyond your control. Instead, figure out the genuine cause of your slip (you let yourself get too hungry; you had junk food in the house) and don't let it happen again (eat more regularly; throw out the junk food). Do not let things go! Initiate action immediately.

Stay Food Wise

So that you can continue to change the shape of your body, it's wise to continue to choose lean proteins, low-starch vegetables, low-sugar carbohydrates, and complex natural carbohydrates as the basis of your diet. Stay away from sugary foods. Sugar and foods that contain it cause an overload of glucose and insulin in your system. Insulin encourages the movement of fat from the bloodstream into fat cells for storage. The cumulative result of these interactions is the ready conversion of simple sugars to body fat. So to fight fat, you must fight the sugar urge. (Exception: If you experience low blood sugar, eating a sugary food immediately can help you in a pinch. For more information on low blood sugar, see appendix A.)

In addition, avoid high-fat foods, such as fried foods, fat-laden snacks, and sweets, since fat has a slowing effect on your metabolism. How much fat your body stores seems to be more closely related to how much fat you eat than to how many calories you eat. In fact, very little of your body fat comes from carbohydrates or protein; most of it comes from fat you eat.

I am frequently asked if it's permissible to eat commercial low-fat or low-carb food products. I am not in favor of doing so—for two important reasons. First, these foods tend to be processed, and compared with natural, clean-burning foods such as lean proteins, vegetables, and fruits, processed foods are like sludge in your system, slowing down your metabolism and contributing little nutrient value to your diet. Second, when fat is removed from foods during the manufacturing process, the food makers usually replace it with some form of sugar and carbohydrate. Some of these foods can wreak havoc on your blood sugar and possibly promote fat storage. However, when you reach maintenance, you can eat almost anything occasionally.

Very important: Continue to eat multiple meals a day to keep your metabolism in a constant state of acceleration. Every time you eat, your metabolic rate increases a little due to the heat that is produced during the digestion and absorption of food. Eating frequently keeps your metabolic furnace stoked and your metabolism speeding along. If you go too long without eating, your metabolism begins to slow.

Just because the 12 days are now over doesn't mean you can go hog wild and eat everything in sight. Continue to practice portion control. Stay aware of what constitutes a serving and don't fudge it by taking more than what's allotted.

Never skip breakfast, either. Read that again: Never skip breakfast. Breakfast is truly the most important meal of the day. Skipping it leads to food cravings later on, intense hunger, and low energy. What's more, research demonstrates that people who regularly eat breakfast keep their weight off; people who don't tend to regain their weight and stay heavy. Eating breakfast is a positive habit that contributes to body-shaping success.

Control Emotional Eating

Many people turn to food when they're down in the dumps—a habit that can pile on the pounds unless you get it under control. Eating lifts the depression—but only temporarily. After the binge, you're apt to feel even worse emotionally because you've overindulged. Guilt-ridden, you can slip into a vicious cycle of overeating and negative emotions.

Emotional eating is a huge problem, particularly among women. One recent national survey by the Calorie Control Council (CCC) found that 36 percent of women blamed weight-loss failures on emotional eating. Other research estimates that 50 to 80 percent of all dieters overeat to relieve depression and other negative emotions. A major problem with emotional eating is the food that is chosen. It's usually high in sugar and processed carbohydrates—"comfort foods" that are easily metabolized into fat.

There are various strategies you can use when you're down in the dumps and want to eat. First, try reaching for low-calorie foods, such as fresh fruit or vegetables or whole grains. Second, as a matter of habit, try to eat more fish. Fish contains beneficial fats that appear to increase levels of neurotransmitters—brain chemicals that transmit messages from one nerve cell to another—particularly serotonin. Serotonin is known as the "happiness neurotransmitter," because elevated levels bring on feelings of tranquility, calm, and emotional well-being. Third, instead of bingeing when you're depressed, be prepared to substitute alternative activities, such as exercise, reading, or other things you enjoy, to take the place of eating. Exercise, in particular, is a great mood booster.

Overcome Plateaus

At first, you'll find yourself losing weight steadily, even rapidly, but at some point this progress will slow and then almost seem to stop altogether. Plateaus like these occur because your body is adjusting to changes, and weight loss slows as a result. Usually, though, plateaus don't hit until several weeks into a diet, so if you experience a plateau, it will occur after you have lost significant pounds and inches. And what's the typical remedy used by many people when this happens? Your instinct may be to either get discouraged and throw in the towel, or drastically reduce your food intake. Neither approach works, of course, and they'll only leave you vulnerable to rebound weight gain. Just keep in mind that your body will plateau. This is natural, but if you stay focused and follow your food plan, you will overcome plateaus.

One of the best defenses against a plateau is regular exercise, particularly a combination of weight training and cardio, as I recommend for the *12-Day Body Shaping Miracle*. Cardio heats up the metabolic activity of your muscles, making your body more efficient at burning fat; resistance training, in addition to developing metabolically active muscle tissue, helps your metabolism stay charged up for as long as 24 hours after your workout. The message here is that if you comply with the recommended exercise methods, you shouldn't have to worry about hitting a plateau. Your progress should be fairly steady.

Also, it's very important to understand the effects of hormones on plateaus. Don't expect to lose any or much weight right before and during your menstrual period. After it stops, you will generally lose weight again.

But if you don't, here is a little-known plateau buster: Make sure you're drinking 100 ounces of water a day, as I emphasize throughout the *12-Day Body Shaping Miracle*. By drinking enough water, you can keep your metabolic fires burning. Studies show that water may contribute to boosting the body's ability to burn more calories, may help reduce your appetite and thus control food intake, and may reduce the amount of dietary fat ultimately stored in the body. Since fat is broken down through a water-involved process called *hydrolysis,* insufficient amounts of water in your body will hinder effective breakdown of fat.

There are other reasons to prioritize water. It helps form the structures of proteins and glycogen, thus strengthening muscles. You can't load muscle cells with glycogen or deliver amino acids to muscle tissue without adequate water. Water plays a key role in digestion, elimination, regulation of body temperature, lubrication of joints, the moisture of your skin, and the maintenance of your muscle tone. It also transports nutrients, oxygen, and glucose to every cell of the body, then removes toxins and impurities from the body. Ironically, if you don't drink enough water, you may store more water, which can show up as extra weight on the scale. This occurs because water dilutes. Without enough water, you may also feel more hungry and tired, lack energy, and become constipated.

Thirst signals the first stage of dehydration. You must stay hydrated and avoid thirst. If you become even slightly dehydrated, you're already behind the curve in your weight-loss efforts. Rehydrate immediately. If you aren't drinking enough water, the signs of dehydration show up in your urine. Darker-colored urine is a sure sign of dehydration, so try to drink enough water to produce clear or pale-yellow-colored urine every two to three hours during the day.

Here's a final tip: When you reach your goal, you can have one to two "cheat" days a week and eat whatever you want, as long as you don't revert to your old habits completely.

Draft Your Body-Shaping Maintenance Plan

The day will come when you'll be wearing clothes that show off the shape of your body. There will be no more avoiding yourself in mirrors . . . no more avoiding shopping for clothes . . . no more dressing to disguise your body . . . no more avoiding being seen naked by your significant other. No more avoidance, period!

When that day arrives, you'll want to have a simple maintenance plan in place. For your final body-shaping assignment, I'd like you to fill out the following sheet and post it where you can see it every single day. Ready? Here goes.

My Maintenance Plan

List the reasons why you do not want to return to your old shape:

_____

_____

_____

_____

_____

List the positive habits you will maintain in order to stay in shape:

_____

_____

_____

_____

_____

List personal danger zones you might face (skipping meals, eating too much late at night, neglecting your workouts, stress-related eating, failing to self-monitor, what have you).

_____

_____

_____

_____

Finally, for each personal danger zone you listed, come up with a strategy or solution that will prevent you from caving in to that particular problem or barrier to maintenance.

_____

_____

_____

_____

You know this already (at least I hope you do): There is a natural feel-good ecstasy associated with having a beautiful, shapely body and showing it off in attractive formfitting clothes. And you'll experience this if you do everything laid out in this book! Decide today and every day that you're through living in an overburdened body; you want to be in one that moves, breathes, and exists in beauty and health.

We've come to the end of this book, but in many ways it's really just the beginning. You now have all the facts, all the basics you need to get in shape and stay there. You have everything you need for a lean, shapely, picture-perfect body for life. Just hang in there, do it, and enjoy the results. You are worth it!

APPENDIX A

Workout and Diet Customizations for Special Medical Conditions

to my readers: Many of you may face special challenges when it comes to losing weight and following a specific workout and eating plan. Please read this section carefully if you have hypoglycemia, diabetes, blood pressure problems, a thyroid condition, digestive disorders, high cholesterol, or dry skin or hair; if you're taking medication; or if you suffer from any type of medical condition. Do your Blueprint, create your exercise routine, and select your custom eating plan, but before beginning, be sure to show the programs to your physician and have him or her make any additional customizations for you and get his or her approval prior to starting. I always advise my clients to *take their makeover program to their doctors* so that they can be fully informed on the diet and exercise issues involved. All of my makeover programs are designed for men and women in normal health, as a way to help them lose weight and become even healthier in the process. All those who have a diagnosed medical condition, or women who are pregnant or trying to get pregnant, should not go on this program or any other weight-reducing or workout program until they have approval from their physician.

Hypoglycemia (Low Blood Sugar)

Has this ever happened to you? You've just finished a workout and you feel drained, weak, tired, or dizzy, or even experience foggy thinking. What is going on? Aren't workouts supposed to energize you? This unsettling incident may be due to a condition called hypoglycemia, or low blood sugar. It occurs when blood levels of *glucose* (blood sugar)—which acts as an energy source for your body—are burned off during exercise and drop too low to fuel your activity. Other chief causes of low blood sugar are insufficient carbohydrates and protein in your bloodstream, and waiting too long between meals.

When there's insufficient glucose in the blood that circulates through your nervous system and other cells, they become energy-starved. Some common symptoms include:

- A cold sweat or blurry vision.
- A feeling of being spaced out, or losing your ability to speak or concentrate.
- feeling lethargic, weak, shaky, or faint.
- Headaches, nausea, or an unexplained hangover.

One way you can prevent hypoglycemia, as well as manage it, is to make sure you eat a carbohydrate and a lean protein prior to exercising, as I recommended in chapter 8. This type of snack helps sustain your glucose flow at a slower rate than would eating a fast carb, which may bring about an immediate demand on insulin to lower the blood sugar and create an even greater drop in blood sugar when you start to exercise. As a further preventive measure, make sure you have a carbohydrate at every meal. If you suffer from any of the above symptoms, ask your physician to administer a glucose tolerance test.

If you experience any symptoms of low blood sugar after just an hour or two without food, chances are you have hypoglycemia, and you should consult your doctor prior to beginning this program.

Hypoglycemia can also cause you to misjudge your hunger. Low glucose levels can make you feel ravenous, and you will reach for anything and everything to remedy the low. At that point, it can be hard to control what you eat. This is when you need to cheat and get your blood sugar normalized. It's okay to eat pie, cake, cheese, or some junk food just to get yourself feeling 100 percent. Then take your food plan to your physician and have him or her adjust it by adding in more carbohydrates.

Generally, though, if you're eating at scheduled times on your custom eating plan, your blood sugar should stay relatively even. But if you still find yourself suffering from low blood sugar, you'll want to tweak your plan to avoid the disturbing symptoms of glucose depletion. In the chart below are some solutions to help you.

IF YOU ARE HYPOGLYCEMIC	
BODY TYPE A	Adjust your eating plan to include a carbohydrate with every meal. This carbohydrate may be a potato or yam (in your designated serving size); an additional serving of grapefruit or berries; or ½ cup of cooked oatmeal. To keep your blood sugar at safe levels, do not skip any meals. As one of your snacks, be sure to eat a carbohydrate such as a yam (6 ounces), or 1 cup of rice and a banana prior to and after your workout. Always include 2 ounces of protein with this carb.
BODY TYPE B	Adjust your eating plan to include a carbohydrate with every meal. This carbohydrate may be brown rice (in your designated serving size), or an additional serving of grapefruit or berries. To keep your blood sugar at safe levels, do not skip any meals. Be sure to eat a carbohydrate and a protein meal prior to and after your workout.
BODY TYPE C	Adjust your eating plan to include a carbohydrate with every meal. This carbohydrate may be brown rice (in your designated serving size), or an additional serving such as a banana or other high-sugar fruit. To keep your blood sugar at safe levels, do not skip any meals. Be sure to eat a carbohydrate and a protein meal prior to and after your workout.
BODY TYPE D	Adjust your eating plan to include a carbohydrate with every meal. This carbohydrate may be brown rice (in your designated serving size). To keep your blood sugar at safe levels, do not skip any meals. Be sure to eat a carbohydrate and a protein meal prior to and after your workout.

BODY TYPE E	Adjust your eating plan to include a carbohydrate with every meal. This carbohydrate may be brown rice or brown rice and beans (in your designated serving size), or a serving of egg whites, oatmeal, or a banana. To keep your blood sugar at safe levels, do not skip any meals. Be sure to eat a carbohydrate and a protein meal prior to and after your workout.

You can further modify the *12-Day Body Shaping Miracle* diet by having fresh pineapple, raisins, or other fruit for snacks during the day, in between meals. Plus, keep energy bars or peanut butter in your office or car in case of a low blood sugar emergency. Should you wind up in such a situation, you'll need to get a simple sugar into your body as quickly as possible. Fruit juice, dried fruits, oranges, or even several jelly beans will help alleviate the symptoms. Waiting too long before eating can be dangerous. You could faint or go into shock. The longer you wait, the more difficult it is to bring your blood sugar back in balance. So don't worry: Cheat with high-sugar foods until you feel 100 percent.

If your symptoms are very severe, eat pie, ice cream, or another high-sugar food. But as soon as you can, consume a slow carbohydrate, which converts to sugar in the body more gradually, along with some lean protein. This combination of foods leads to a more even blood sugar level and more sustained energy. Never eat protein by itself; this will drive your blood sugar even lower.

Most of us will experience low blood sugar at some point or another, so it's important to know the symptoms and how to handle them. If you are extremely hypoglycemic, however, you may need to add a carbohydrate to every one of your meals. Also, have a carb and a protein after your workout too. Make sure your physician helps you customize your diet.

High Blood Pressure (Hypertension)

Largely a symptomless disease, high blood pressure affects one in four Americans. Normal blood pressure is equal to or less than 120 over 80 most of the time. The top number refers to *systolic* pressure, the pressure in the artery when the heart contracts; the lower number refers to *diastolic* pressure, the pressure in the artery when the heart relaxes. Every incremental hike in blood pressure corresponds to a rise in your risk of heart attack, heart failure, stroke, and kidney disease.

Exercise can have a positive effect on your blood pressure. For 30 to 120 minutes after performing cardio exercise, your blood pressure tends to lower or stabilize in a normal range. Research shows that if you continue to make exercising a regular part of your lifestyle, over time it can help you reduce and even maintain more normal blood pressure.

The American College of Sports Medicine states that you can effectively lower your blood pressure with moderate-intensity exercise performed three to five times a week for 20 to 60 minutes per session. In fact, moderate-intensity exercise such as brisk walking may have an even greater blood-pressure-lowering effect than higher-intensity training (like running).

The ACSM does not recommend resistance training as the sole form of exercise if you have high blood pressure, since it does not appear to be as effective in lowering blood pressure as aerobic exercise. In fact, performing resistance training will increase your blood pressure, so it is vital that you follow your physician's protocol for managing hypertension, as well as doing aerobic exercise along with resistance training.

How exactly does regular exercise lower your blood pressure? Although the jury is still out on this question, exercise does appear to relax your blood vessels, decrease the levels of certain hormones in your body, and improve kidney function—all situations that contribute to good blood pressure control.

If you have been diagnosed with high blood pressure, regular exercise as recommended on this program should help you, since a couch-potato lifestyle is associated with increased blood pressure and is a major risk factor for cardiovascular disease. Your custom eating plan should also help you considerably, since it is very low in sodium, one of the chief instigators of high blood pressure. Low-sodium diets do a lot to nudge your blood pressure down, and every little bit of pressure lowering helps. Losing weight also helps get your blood pressure back into the safety zone.

With high blood pressure, however, you may want to eliminate egg whites (if your eating plan calls for them)—they are very high in sodium. You may substitute another source of protein for the egg whites, such as fish or lean poultry. Diets that are well populated with fish somehow seem to counteract high blood pressure.

Also, make sure you review your workout and eating plan with your doctor, particularly if you are taking blood pressure medication. Even after following your eating plan for just 12 days, your blood pressure may drop naturally, and your doctor may then need to adjust your medication.

Low Blood Pressure (Hypotension)

When you exercise, certain changes take place in your cardiovascular system. One of the greatest changes is due to the blood flow diverted to your exercising muscles. When such a large increase in blood flow heads to muscles, there can be a drop in blood pressure. Generally, this drop is normal and beneficial, but in anyone who is susceptible to low blood pressure it can increase the risk of fainting.

In some cases, people who lose fluid through sweating, diarrhea, or vomiting can experience low blood pressure, since these conditions reduce blood volume. Other causes may be dehydration or the loss of electrolytes (minerals) and sodium through perspiration and exercise. As I mentioned earlier, if you're taking blood pressure medication, particularly diuretics, you can experience low blood pressure.

Normal blood pressure is 120/80 or lower. Unlike high blood pressure, there are no clear-cut standards for the diagnosis of low blood pressure, although many physicians consider a reading of 105/70 to 100/60 to be hypotensive. If your doctor says your blood pressure is unusually low, this should be evaluated medically, since low blood pressure isn't a specific disease but rather the sign of some underlying medical problem. There are telltale symptoms of low blood pressure, however, and these include:

- Fatigue, malaise, lethargy, or a general sleepiness
- Irregular or elevated heart rate

- Clammy or sweaty skin
- Dizziness or light-headedness

With low blood pressure, you need some sodium. That being the case, add a little salt to your diet, particularly in the morning. No-sodium-added canned tuna and low-sodium soy sauce are two excellent ways to incorporate some sodium into your diet without triggering too much water retention. If you suffer from symptoms of low blood pressure, try to have a source of salt on hand at all times. Carrying a few salt packets in your pocket is a good solution. Consume one right away if you start to feel dizzy or light-headed. In addition, you can eat a salty snack such as potato chips with something sugary like orange juice. This salt-sugar combination can help stabilize blood pressure. Another good move you can make is to replenish lost electrolytes and sodium with a supplement such as Emergen-C or Gatorade in order to elevate your blood pressure to more normal levels. In fact, you can mix salt packets into Gatorade, and this combination will rapidly normalize low blood pressure. Losing weight or reducing carbohydrates in your snacks can lower blood pressure. Taking your blood pressure regularly is important. In fact, it can be necessary if you have abnormal blood pressure. In addition, make sure your doctor reviews your customized eating plan and workout routine.

Diabetes

Diabetes is a blood sugar metabolism disorder in which there is too much sugar (glucose) circulating in the blood. With diabetes, two things go wrong. First, the body might not be making any or enough insulin. Second, the cells may not respond properly to insulin and thus receive no nourishment, since insulin helps usher nutrients into cells. In both situations, glucose starts building up in the bloodstream, and this provokes all sorts of metabolic problems. Your body becomes starved of energy, and eventually its organs can deteriorate unless blood sugar can be brought under control. Diabetes is thus a serious, potentially life-threatening disease that must be medically monitored and treated.

One of the ways to control blood sugar is through exercise, which has been shown to lower your blood sugar level. Exercise also reduces your risk of heart disease, which is common in people who have diabetes. If you have been diagnosed with diabetes, you should talk to your physician about what exercise is right for you. Many doctors recommend aerobic exercise, such as walking, jogging, and bicycling—all of which help you manage your weight (being overweight complicates diabetes), help you breathe more deeply, and make your heart work harder. Resistance training is also very beneficial. It encourages insulin use by activating a key protein in muscle cells that helps insulin push glucose into these cells. A caution: If you have problems with the nerves in your feet or legs, as many people with diabetes do, your doctor may want to limit you to low-impact exercises that don't aggravate your feet, such as using a stationary bicycle.

There may be some risks if you have diabetes and follow an exercise program. The benefits, however, outweigh the risks. One risk is that your blood sugar can become too low (hypoglycemia) after you exercise. For this reason, it is vital that you check your blood sugar level before and after exercising. (Your physician can give you guidelines on what your glucose level should be before you exercise.) Have a snack handy in case your blood sugar level drops during or after exercise. If your glucose level is too low or too high before you exercise, you should not start your workout until the level improves.

If you are overweight and have type 2 diabetes (also called non-insulin-dependent diabetes mellitus or NIDDM), weight loss through diet and regular exercise can be essential to controlling the disease. In many cases, losing weight makes it possible for people with type 2 diabetes to discontinue taking medication altogether. Weight loss may also reduce cholesterol and blood pressure, both of which are commonly elevated in this form of the disease.

Because your custom eating plan, in conjunction with diabetes medications, may lower your blood sugar, it is important to carry glucose tablets with you in case you suffer a hypoglycemic emergency.

Even though this eating plan and your workout can help regulate blood sugar in people with diabetes, you should not begin this program without consulting your doctor first, particularly if you require supplemental insulin.

Ulcers and Other Digestive Disorders

Digestive troubles plague millions of Americans and can be made worse by offending foods. With problems such as ulcers, you'll want to identify foods that aggravate the problem, then course-correct nutritionally and with other lifestyle measures, under the guidance of your physician. Here are a few general pointers:

- Follow a balanced diet that focuses on whole, unprocessed foods, such as those I recommend on this program, as opposed to substances that trigger digestive distress. Some of the most common offenders are fatty foods and milk products (both of which stimulate acid release), caffeinated beverages, coffee (regular and decaf), chocolate, vinegar, black pepper, and chili powder.
- Be defensive in your food preparation. Avoid raw vegetables and instead cook your vegetables to help break them down and make it easier for your body to digest. Eat whipped or mashed potatoes, if your eating plan prescribes them. In addition, eat very light fish (such as sole or flounder), ground turkey breast, and egg whites, where your eating plan calls for these foods.
- Practice stress-control measures. What medical experts do know about the link between stress and ulcers is that stress may aggravate them or bring them on prematurely. You can reduce your stress by regularly practicing Abdominal Breathing, regular exercise, and relaxation activities such as meditation.

If you suffer from inflammatory bowel disease (IBD), such as Crohn's disease, or ulcerative colitis or other digestive disorders like diverticulosis or spastic colon, always consult your physician prior to changing your diet.

Thyroid Disease

Straddling your windpipe is a bow-tie-shaped mass of tissue called the thyroid gland. It produces specific hormones that set your metabolic tempo. If that tempo is slow—a condition called hypothyroidism or underactive thyroid—your thyroid gland may not be producing enough hormones and your body's food-handling ability is compromised. Instead of being converted into energy, food is mostly stockpiled as body fat.

Thyroid disease can thus affect your weight loss. When your thyroid is underactive, difficulty losing weight, or continued weight gain, can be traced to a drop in the metabolism that frequently accompanies hypothyroidism. Even after your hypothyroidism is properly treated with medication, you may find that your metabolism has not bounced back to where it was before. There are some additional measures you can take, and these are listed below. Talk to your physician about whether any of these actions can help you.

- *Eat breakfast.* As I have pointed out in this book, not eating breakfast can slow your metabolism. Without enough nourishment to start the day, your body goes into a temporary starvation mode, thinking it isn't going to be fed, and consequently it starts hoarding fat for survival. Avoiding this reaction is as simple as starting the day with a nutritious meal. People who regularly eat breakfast have an easier time losing weight and keeping it off.

- *Eat multiple meals throughout the day.* Having frequent meals, as I advise on all my makeover diets, keeps your blood sugar stable, rekindles your metabolism, and provides a steady source of fuel to drive your metabolism.

- *Perform moderate cardio exercise.* This form of exercise provides a real boost to metabolism. Keep it moderate. People with thyroid disease are often suffering from fatigue. Exercising too strenuously for too long can aggravate thyroid-related fatigue.

- *Include resistance training.* This form of exercise develops firm, strong muscles, which are metabolically active. This means they can burn body fat more efficiently than untoned muscle, even at rest. The more lean muscle you develop, the more fat you can burn.

- *Don't neglect water.* The energy-using process of metabolism needs sufficient water every day to work efficiently. Drink your 100 ounces (roughly 12 cups) of water daily.

If you are eating according to your plan and still find you have trouble losing weight, it may be a good idea to see your physician and request a thyroid function test. This test checks your blood to determine whether levels of thyroid hormones fall within a normal range. If you are diagnosed with an underactive thyroid, it can be treated and corrected with prescription thyroid medication.

Pregnant or Nursing

Many women have questions and concerns about exercising during pregnancy and while nursing. Although you should discuss these issues with your physician, medical experts generally agree that exercise —within certain limits—can be beneficial. If you are pregnant, exercise may help you feel less fatigued, boost your energy level, and help you better deal with the physical demands of labor and recovery in the postpartum period. Of course, no woman should start an exercise program during pregnancy.

Your physician can advise you as to whether you can continue your regular exercise program during your entire pregnancy. Some women, however, may have to discontinue exercising due to medical conditions such as obesity, diabetes, orthopedic limitations, or obstetric complications. If you exercise while pregnant and experience any unusual symptoms, stop immediately and see your physician right away. Some of these symptoms include vaginal bleeding, dizziness, headache, chest pain, muscle weakness, pain or swelling, and fluid leakage.

The American College of Obstetricians and Gynecologists (ACOG) stresses that where no complications exist, 30 minutes or more of moderate exercise a day on most, if not all days of the week, is recommended for pregnant women. As for resistance training, talk to your physician—it may not be appropriate for all pregnant women. I can't emphasize it enough: Get your physician's approval before starting or continuing an exercise program.

Do not follow the *12-Day Body Shaping Miracle* eating plan if you are pregnant or nursing. Your body requires extra calories at this time. Save this program until you've stopped nursing. It can be a great tool for shedding postpregnancy pounds in a hurry.

Menopause

Many women still take estrogen in the form of birth control pills or hormone replacement therapy with estrogen, progesterone, or both. Estrogen can promote water retention. This does not mean, however, that you cannot lose weight. It just means that you may lose it more slowly, in general. Some good news, though: The *12-Day Body Shaping Miracle* has proven an effective tool for women in menopause who need to kick-start their fat-burning mechanisms, despite taking supplemental estrogen.

Food Allergies

Food allergies can be a hidden cause of weight gain, and the usual suspects provoking reactions in susceptible people are milk, eggs, peanuts, soy foods, wheat, fish, and shellfish. If you know you're allergic to certain foods, don't eat them! Working with your physician, identify alternatives that you can tolerate.

You're not alone if you have found out that you should leave wheat and foods containing it off your plate. Although sometimes diagnosed as a wheat allergy, celiac sprue disease is really an inherited genetic disorder that affects 1 in every 300 people. If you have this disease, you cannot eat the protein (or gluten) found in wheat, rye, barley, and, to a lesser extent, oats. For people with celiac sprue disease, eating gluten sets off an autoimmune response that causes damage to the small intestine, which in turn loses its ability to absorb nutrients from food into the body.

Check with your health food store for information on wheat-free and gluten-free products (foods labeled wheat-free are not necessarily gluten-free). As you plan your nutrition, it is important for you to focus on the foods you can eat, rather than what you cannot. People with food allergies should work with their physician, or a registered dietitian, to ensure good nutritional health.

High Cholesterol

Cholesterol has somewhat of a split personality in the body, with a good side because it's required for digesting dietary fats, making hormones, building cell walls, and other important processes. But cholesterol also has a bad side. Too much of the wrong type of circulating cholesterol (LDL cholesterol) can injure arteries and cause heart attacks and stroke.

Cholesterol levels are checked with a blood test. Your total blood cholesterol will fall into one of these categories:

Desirable—less than 200 mg/dL
Borderline high risk—200–239 mg/dL
High risk—240 mg/dL and over

Your LDL cholesterol will fall into one of these categories:

Optimum—less than 100 mg/dL
Near/above optimum—100–129 mg/dL
Borderline high—130–159 mg/dL
High—160–189 mg/dL
Very high—190 mg/dL and above

Your LDL cholesterol level greatly affects your risk of heart attack and stroke. The lower your LDL cholesterol, the lower your risk. In fact, it's a better gauge of risk than total blood cholesterol.

As for HDL cholesterol (dubbed the "good kind"), in the average woman, healthy values range from 50 to 60 mg/dL. With this number, the higher, the better. HDL cholesterol that is less than 40 mg/dL is considered low and puts you at high risk for heart disease. HDL helps prevent a cholesterol buildup in blood vessels.

Regular physical activity is one lifestyle measure you can take to help control cholesterol problems. According to research, resistance training, in particular, may improve cholesterol level by decreasing LDL cholesterol levels and increasing HDL cholesterol levels.

If you have high cholesterol, avoid red meat and shellfish, regardless of what body type you have. The saturated fat and dietary cholesterol in these foods contribute to high cholesterol in the blood, which in turn clogs blood vessels and increases your risk of heart attack and stroke. For protein, stick with lean poultry and fish instead. Switching from one or two large meals per day to five or six smaller ones can lower total cholesterol by approximately 5 percent, according to a study at the University of Cambridge in England. Finally, make sure you review your eating plan and exercise routine with your doctor.

Dry Skin or Hair

If your skin or hair is unusually dry, add a little more fat to your diet. There are ways to do this without destroying your fat loss. For example, add about a teaspoon of flaxseed oil to your salad. Or you can substitute a more fatty fish such as salmon, trout, or sea bass for one of your proteins. If you do this, eliminate the carbohydrate at that meal and substitute extra greens instead. Here's why: Additional fat taken with carbohydrates has the unfortunate consequence of being more readily stored. Eliminating the carb will prevent this from happening and keep your weight loss on target. Plus, the fat in the fish or flaxseed oil helps sustain your glucose levels so that your blood sugar doesn't plummet too much from lack of carbs. Obviously, be extremely cautious about this sort of dietary manipulation if you are prone to hypoglycemia.

On Any Medication

You may be surprised to learn that there are more than 100 prescription medications with the common side effect of weight gain. Some of the worst offenders are antidepressants, blood pressure drugs, steroids, diabetic medicines, hormone replacement therapy, and anti-seizure medications. If you are taking any of these drugs or others, talk with your doctor about whether they may interfere with your desire to lose weight. Never discontinue taking a drug or adjust your dosage without first consulting with your doctor.

In addition, some foods interact adversely with medications (grapefruit and grapefruit juice are two examples), so make sure your physician is familiar with your eating plan and can review it before you start your body makeover.

APPENDIX B

Additional Resources

Food and Nutrition Information

CalorieKing, at www.calorieking.com, is a searchable database with nutritional information on more than 30,000 generic and brand-name foods, including more than 150 fast-food chains.

Continuum Health Partners, Inc., features a fiber content chart at www.weheal ny.org/healthinfo/dietaryfiber/fibercontentchart.html. The foods are organized by fiber and calorie content; the list includes foods with no fiber.

Resistance Training

The Web site of the American College of Sports Medicine (ACSM) (www.acsm.org) offers information on resistance training, working out at home or at an exercise facility, selecting a personal trainer, and more. The ACSM advances and integrates scientific research to provide educational and practical applications of exercise science and sports medicine.

The National Strength and Conditioning Association (NSCA) certifies personal trainers. For help in finding one, log on to www.nsca-lift.org. The NSCA also has online articles covering all aspects of strength and conditioning.

Information on Medical Conditions

If you suffer from any of the conditions listed in appendix A, learn more about your treatment options by logging on to www.webmd.com. WebMD provides valuable health information, tools for managing your health, and support to those who seek information.

Michael Thurmond's Makeover Programs

Log on to www.provida.com for information on additional tools to make over your body and stay motivated. There is also information on my Living Lean maintenance program so that you can keep your body at your goal weight.

If you need to lose weight rapidly but safely for an upcoming event such as a class reunion, wedding, important date, or vacation—or just fit into a dress that's now too snug—refer to my book *6-Day Body Makeover*, which is available wherever books are sold. This is an *accelerated* six-day diet designed to let you drop a whole dress or pant size in just under a week, without starving.

Also available is *Makeover America Cookbook,* which gives you nearly 150 mouthwatering and approved recipes that can help you prepare your food deliciously on the *12-Day Body Shaping Miracle.* Enjoy foods from BBQ Meatballs to Butter Rum Baked Apples . . . you won't believe it's fat-loss food! This cookbook is available through www.provida.com.

If you purchase the *6-Week Body Makeover* program, you can get the answers you need, on the phone or online, from one of my specially trained *6-Week Body Makeover* specialists. This assistance is available 24 hours a day and includes a recipe database, success stories, and nutritional research updates.

Also available 24 hours a day is an online support community. In this supportive forum you can ask questions, get answers, share stories, and get motivated.

Additional information is available at www.bodymakeover.com or www.mybodymakeover.com.

APPENDIX C

Scientific References

a portion of the information in this book comes from medical research reports in both popular and scientific publications, Internet sources, and computer searches of medical databases of research abstracts.

Chapter 1. The Shape of Things to Come

Canoy, D., et al. 2005. Cigarette smoking and fat distribution in 21,828 British men and women: a population-based study. *Obesity Research* 13: 1466–1475.

Oregon Health & Science University. 2005. OHSU researchers uncover cause, possible treatment for abdominal fat in postmenopausal women. News release, June 6.

Chapter 3. Master the Mind–Body Connection

Epel, E. S., et al. 2000. Stress and body shape: Stress-induced cortisol secretion is consistently greater among women with central fat. *Psychosomatic Medicine* 62: 623–632.

University of California–San Francisco. 2000. An assessment of yourself as rich and powerful may keep you healthy, according to UCSF study. News release, November 19.

Chapter 4. How to Reshape Your Body in 12 Days

Carter, R., et al. 1988. Exercise conditioning in the rehabilitation of patients with chronic obstructive pulmonary disease. *Archives of Physical Medicine and Rehabilitation* 69: 118–122.

McDougall, J., et al. 1995. Rapid reduction of serum cholesterol and blood pressure by a twelve-day, very low fat, strictly vegetarian diet. *Journal of the American College of Nutrition* 14: 491–496.

Sonka, J., et al. 1991. Hormonal, metabolic and cardiovascular response to the duration of a combined slimming regimen. *Czech Medicine* 14: 156–163.

Chapter 7. Cardio Meltdown

Kohrt, W. M., et al. 1992. Exercise training improves fat distribution patterns in 60- to 70-year-old men and women. *Journal of Gerontology* 47: M99–M105.

Rodin, J., et al. 1990. Weight cycling and fat distribution. *International Journal of Obesity* 14: 303–310.

Chapter 8. My Figure-Shaping Nutrition Plan

Barlow, J. 2001. Consuming more protein, fewer carbohydrates may be healthier. Press release, News Bureau, University of Illinois at Urbana-Champaign.

Burke, L. M. 1997. Nutrition for post-exercise recovery. *Australian Journal of Science and Medicine in Sport* 1: 3–10.

Clark, N. 1992. Fluid facts: what, when, and how much to drink. *The Physician and Sportsmedicine* 20: 33–36.

Editor. 1992. Alcohol and weight gain—a double whammy. *Medical Update* 16: 4.

Howarth, N. C., et al. 2001. Dietary fiber and weight regulation. *Nutrition Review* 59: 129–139.

Ivy, J. L. 1998. Glycogen resynthesis after exercise: effect of carbohydrate intake. *International Journal of Sports Medicine* 19: S142–S145.

Kleiner, S. M. 1999. Water: an essential but overlooked nutrient. *Journal of the American Dietetic Association* 99: 200–206.

LeBlanc, J., et al. 1993. Components of postprandial thermogenesis in relation to meal frequency in humans. *Canadian Journal of Physiology and Pharmacology* 71: 879–883.

Maffucci, D. M., et al. 2000. Towards optimizing the timing of the pre-exercise meal. *International Journal of Sports Nutrition and Exercise Metabolism* 10: 103–113.

Epilogue: Beyond the First 12 Days: Look Better than Ever, Forever

Bouchard, C., et al. 1990. Long-term exercise training with constant energy intake: effect on body composition and selected metabolic variables. *International Journal of Obesity* 14: 57–73.

Kayman, S., et al. 1990. Maintenance and relapse after weight loss in women: behavioral aspects. *American Journal of Clinical Nutrition* 52: 800–807.

Wing, R. R., et al. 2001. Successful weight loss maintenance. *Annual Review of Nutrition* 21: 323–341.

Wyatt, H. R., et al. 2002. Long-term weight loss and breakfast in subjects in the National Weight Control Registry. *Obesity Research* 10: 78–82.

Appendix A: Workout and Diet Customizations for Special Medical Conditions

White, J., 1992. Exercising for two: what's safe for the active pregnant woman? *The Physician and Sportsmedicine* 20: 179–186.

INDEX

NOTE: *Italic page numbers* indicate photographs

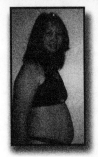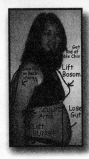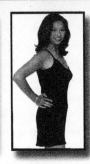
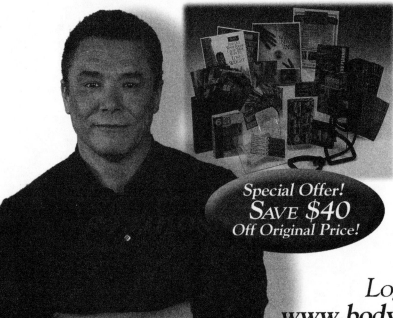